Environmental Health Literacy Update - New Evidence, Methodologies and Perspectives

Edited by Rafael Moreno-Gómez-Toledano

Published in London, United Kingdom

Environmental Health Literacy Update - New Evidence, Methodologies and Perspectives
http://dx.doi.org/10.5772/intechopen.111125
Edited by Rafael Moreno-Gómez-Toledano

Contributors
Rafael Moreno-Gómez-Toledano, Clara Jabal-Uriel, Michael Greenberg, Henry Mayer, David Kosson, Timothy Fields, Zemachu Ashuro, Gose Husen Washo, Kuma Diriba, Benjamin Mwangi, Lutendo Sylvia Mudau, Ayanda Myranda Derby Thumbathi, Davies Veli Nkosi, Dominic Halsmer, Domenica Baez

First published in London, United Kingdom, 2024 by IntechOpen
IntechOpen is the global imprint of INTECHOPEN LIMITED, registered in England and Wales, registration number: 11086078, 167-169 Great Portland Street, London, W1W 5PF, United Kingdom

British Library Cataloguing-in-Publication Data
A catalogue record for this book is available from the British Library

Additional hard and PDF copies can be obtained from orders@intechopen.com

Environmental Health Literacy Update - New Evidence, Methodologies and Perspectives
Edited by Rafael Moreno-Gómez-Toledano
p. cm.
Print ISBN 978-1-83769-766-3
Online ISBN 978-1-83769-765-6
eBook (PDF) ISBN 978-1-83769-770-0

For EU product safety concerns:
IN TECH d.o.o., Prolaz Marije Krucifikse Kozulić 3, 51000 Rijeka, Croatia,
info@intechopen.com or visit our website at intechopen.com.

Meet the editor

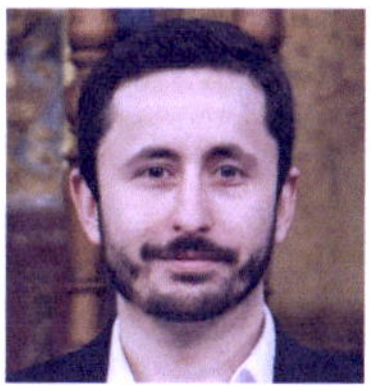

Rafael Moreno-Gómez-Toledano specializes in endocrine disruptors. Most of his research career has focused on investigating the impacts of bisphenol A (BPA) on the renal and cardiovascular systems. This paradigm encompasses chronic kidney disease and diabetic nephropathy in the renal context, as well as cellular senescence and necroptosis of the vascular endothelium. His latest work has identified new associations between emerging bisphenols that replace BPA (such as BPF or BPS) and diabetes, renal, and cardiovascular pathologies. Subsequently, he worked on creating bioinformatic models for analyzing miRNA targets in cardiovascular pathologies at the Ramón y Cajal Hospital, Spain. Currently, he is a professor of Human Anatomy and Embryology at the University of Alcalá, Spain.

Contents

Preface

Over the past century, we have experienced unparalleled technological development, unlike any other time in human history. While this is exceptional, it has underlying issues. Technological advancements have resulted in significant global changes at various levels. Some changes are highly evident, such as deforestation, ecosystem alteration (or destruction), species extinction, and shifts in planetary temperature. Others are less apparent but of great importance to public health, including the release of endocrine disruptors, exposure to pesticides, or the ingestion of microplastics. Consequently, environmental health literacy has become necessary for the global population. This book gathers new evidence, methodologies, and perspectives to update the paradigm and enhance the lives of the general population as well as future generations.

This book explores new evidence, methodologies, and perspectives regarding environmental health literacy through the combined insights of authors from different countries and academic and health institutions. In this way, issues of paramount importance to global health, such as the impact of monomers used in plastics on child health, a group susceptible to endocrine disruptors, are addressed. Similarly, the need to conduct environmental studies related to microplastic pollution represents a crucial and recently discovered turning point. Furthermore, new online databases to identify environmental justice issues, a matter of great global relevance, are also explored. Additionally, the book presents three exciting studies focusing on issues in emerging countries, such as air quality in hospitals, communicable diseases, and urban waste problems. Finally, the book concludes with a perspectives chapter, applying a novel Affordance-based Reverse Systems Engineering approach.

I sincerely thank all the authors who have participated in this book, contributing their unique perspectives on environmental health literacy, which is essential in the current social context. Firstly, I thank Dr. Clara Jabal-Uriel for co-authoring the chapter dedicated to microplastics and pollinators with me. I hope that future research endeavors contribute to resolving the issue for the betterment of global health. I also want to thank Elisa Moreno-Mizileanu for her indispensable logistical support and Elvira Baumgartner, who has done a fantastic job coordinating and managing the book. Without her and the IntechOpen publishing company, this book would not have been created. Continuing with expressions of gratitude, I extend my heartfelt thanks to all the co-authors who have contributed to this book. Each of you has played a crucial role in creating a comprehensive and insightful exploration of environmental health literacy. Your collective contributions, dedication, and experience have greatly enriched the content and depth of this work. As a result, we can move in the right direction, a path that will positively impact future generations' health in a global context where environmental health significantly affects society.

Rafael Moreno-Gómez-Toledano
Department of Surgery, Medical and Social Sciences,
University of Alcalá,
Alcalá de Henares, Spain

Chapter 1

Introductory Chapter: The Significance of Environmental Health Literacy – Children and BPA-free Plastics

Rafael Moreno-Gómez-Toledano

1. Introduction

Over the past century, there has been unparalleled technological development, unlike any other time in human history. While this is exceptional, it is not without underlying issues. The result of technological advancement has led to significant changes at various levels across the globe. Some of these changes are highly evident, such as deforestation, ecosystem alteration (or destruction), species extinction, and shifts in planetary temperature, while others are less apparent but of great importance to public health, such as the release of endocrine disruptors, exposure to pesticides, or the ingestion of microplastics. These are a few examples of the human impact on the planet.

Some authors have begun to use the term Anthropocene to define this new era in the planet's history, during which humans have become a global force that has pushed the planet beyond its natural boundaries [1]. For the first time in the last 24,000 years, there are temperature changes occurring, with an increase of 1.1°C above pre-industrial levels and a current rate of 0.2°C per decade [2]. The significant consequence of the Anthropocene is the exponential increase in potential risks to human health. Therefore, environmental health literacy (EHL) is a fundamental concept and a necessity for the modern era.

In simple terms, Environmental Health Literacy (EHL) can be defined as the understanding that environmental exposures can impact health [3]. Delving deeper into the concept, it is the ability to seek, comprehend, assess, and use environmental health information to make more informed decisions and reduce health risks [4]. EHL is a field of study that integrates components from various disciplines, including health literacy, risk communication, environmental health, communication research, and safety culture [5]. In 2016, the World Health Organization estimated that 24% of global deaths were caused by environmental factors such as water and air pollution, radiation, workplace hazards, noise, climate change, and issues related to water and agricultural practices. For children under the age of 5, the percentage of deaths related to environmental factors rises to 28% [6].

Children under the age of 5 represent a particularly sensitive population in modern society, as they are exposed to numerous xenobiotic elements even before birth. Elements as commonplace as tobacco smoke increase the risk of sudden infant death in the first year of life [7, 8]. It is important to note that two-thirds of deaths related to environmental factors occur in underdeveloped countries due to pathologies stemming from air and water pollution [9]. However, there are issues that occur across the globe, such as exposure to endocrine disruptors resulting from the use and consumption of plastic materials.

Within the range of monomers associated with the plastic industry, one of the most prominent in recent years is bisphenol A (BPA). BPA is a phenolic compound that is widely distributed due to its multiple uses as a monomer, additive, and plasticizer in plastic polymer production [10]. This compound can be found in a multitude of everyday items, such as food containers, toys, dental fillings, medical-surgical materials, or even clothing [11–16]. Its significance, apart from being influenced by its versatility and productivity, lies in its ability to modulate the action of estrogen receptors. BPA is known as one of the primary endocrine disruptors currently under scrutiny by the scientific community.

Due to the heterogeneous distribution of BPA, the potential magnitude and impact it can have on the population are a cause for concern. In recent years, a plastic recycling system has been developed that categorizes plastics into seven categories. In most everyday plastic items, you can identify a triangle with a number from 1 to 7 inside. This coding system was created by the Plastics Industry Association [17] and was recently improved in collaboration with the American Society for Testing and Materials (ASTM), resulting in the current voluntary consensus standard ASTM D7611 [18]. This standard includes the following categories: (1) polyethylene terephthalate (PET); (2) high-density polyethylene (HDPE); (3) polyvinyl chloride (PVC); (4) low-density polyethylene (LDPE); (5) polypropylene (PP); (6) polystyrene (PS); (7) other (materials made from more than one resin from categories 1 to 6) [19].

It is common in academic literature to find texts that describe BPA as the primary monomer used in the production of polycarbonate, a plasticizer in the synthesis of epoxy resins, and an additive in the manufacturing of PVC (codes 3 and 7) [11, 20]. Even though it can be used as an additive in various types of plastics, the possibility of its presence in other materials is usually not considered. In fact, there are numerous online spaces where it is claimed that certain polymers are harmful, while others are considered to pose no potential health risks. These sources often reinforce these axioms with information from the media. Consequently, it is common to come across statements emphasizing the safety of plastics categorized in groups 1, 2, 4, and 5, while those in categories 3, 6, and 7 are considered dangerous to health [21–23]. However, there is evidence in academic literature that BPA is present in all elements of the plastic classification system [24–29]. Given all that has been discussed, environmental health literacy is crucial so that the population can understand the magnitude of the problem and can take measures to reduce exposure to these types of monomers, with special attention to the most vulnerable population groups: newborns and children.

In recent years, there has also been a growing trend of producing items for children with the “BPA-free” label in response to the evidence indicating the potential hazards of BPA, especially in these vulnerable population groups [30]. However, the removal of BPA from plastic synthesis may not necessarily lead to an improvement in health if the substitute molecules exert the same deleterious effects as BPA itself. When conducting a quick internet search for images of “BPA-free” labels, one can find various designs with different fonts, but most of them feature one or more plant leaves, which conveys a sense of "natural" to the buyer. In other cases, terms like "non-toxic," "all-natural," "safe," "clean," or "healthy" may be seen. However, are these claims supported by scientific evidence?

In academic literature, it has been described that in "BPA-free" products, BPA has been replaced with molecules that could have similar physiological effects, such as bisphenol S or F (BPS or BPF, respectively) [31]. These molecules have not been extensively studied, but there are already concerning pieces of evidence about their potential effects on children. To provide some examples, a positive association has been observed between BPF and the risk of obesity in children and adolescents [32], as well as associations between BPS and BPF with asthma and/or fever [33]. There have also been descriptions that both substitute molecules could have a similar endocrine-disrupting capacity to BPA, as shown in a study conducted on children and adolescents [34].

Furthermore, there are alarming indications of the possible impact of BPA substitute molecules on cognitive and neurological development. For instance, Bornehag et al. [35] found a significant association between prenatal exposure to BPF and the cognitive function of 7-year-old children. Jiang et al. [36] provided evidence that prenatal exposure to BPA and BPS could affect neurological development in children. Kim et al. [37] even determined an association between BPS and BPF with attention-deficit/hyperactivity disorder in 6-year-old children. Therefore, it is of utmost importance to increase efforts in EHL simultaneously with the implementation of governmental measures to minimize exposure to these compounds.

2. Conclusions

Today, environmental health literacy is becoming increasingly important for public health because we are living in a new era with a growing number of potential environmental hazards. The population should have reliable and scientifically validated information about the potential environmental hazards they may face. Furthermore, in the case of children under 5 years of age, a group with a particular susceptibility to endocrine disruptors, obtaining information and implementing regulations should be a priority.

Acknowledgements

The author wants to thank Dr. Ricardo J. Bosch for his significant contribution to both professional and personal development, without which the completion of this chapter would not have been possible—additionally, special thanks to Elisa Moreno-Mizileanu for her indispensable logistical support.

Conflict of interest

The author declares no conflict of interest.

Author details

Rafael Moreno-Gómez-Toledano
Department of Biological Systems/Physiology, Universidad de Alcalá,
Alcalá de Henares, Spain

*Address all correspondence to: r.morenogomeztoledano@gmail.com

References

[1] Olff M. Crises in the anthropocene. European Journal of Psychotraumatology. 2023;**14**:2170818

[2] Tong S, Samet JM, Steffen W, et al. Solidarity for the anthropocene. Environmental Research. 2023;**235**: 116716

[3] Rohlman D, Kile ML, Irvin VL. Developing a short assessment of environmental health literacy (SA-EHL). International Journal of Environmental Research and Public Health. 2022;**19**: 2062

[4] Raufman J, Blansky D, Lounsbury DW, et al. Environmental health literacy and household air pollution-associated symptoms in Kenya: A cross-sectional study. Environmental Health. 2020;**19**:89

[5] Lindsey M, Chen SR, Ben R, et al. Defining environmental health literacy. International Journal of Environmental Research and Public Health. 2021;**18**:11626

[6] Bert F, Gea M, Previti C, et al. The environmental health literacy of Italian general population: The SPeRA cross-sectional study. International Journal of Environmental Research and Public Health. 2023;**20**:4486

[7] Ministerio de Sanidad - Ciudadanos - Salud y Medio Ambiente. Available from: https://www.sanidad.gob.es/ciudadanos/saludAmbLaboral/medioAmbiente/home2.htm [Accessed: September 19, 2023]

[8] Tobacco and sudden infant death syndrome (SIDS) - Canada.ca. Available from: https://www.canada.ca/en/health-canada/services/health-concerns/tobacco/legislation/tobacco-product-labelling/smoking-sudden-infant-death-syndrome.html [Accessed: September 19, 2023]

[9] Ortega-García JA, Tellerías L, Ferrís-Tortajada J, et al. Amenazas, desafíos y oportunidades para la salud medioambiental pediátrica en Europa, América Latina y el Caribe. Anales de Pediatría. 2019;**90**:124.e1-124.e11

[10] Moreno-Gómez-Toledano R. Relationship between emergent BPA-substitutes and renal and cardiovascular diseases in adult population. Environmental Pollution. 2021;**313**:120106

[11] Vandenberg LN, Hauser R, Marcus M, et al. Human exposure to bisphenol A (BPA). Reproductive Toxicology. 2007;**24**:139-177

[12] Moreno-Gomez-Toledano R, Arenas IM, Velez-Velez E, Bosch RJ. New evidence for a role of Bisphenol A in cell integrity. Implications in the human population. BIOCELL. 2021;**46**(2):305-308

[13] Dursun E, Fron-Chabouis HH, Attal J-PP, et al. Bisphenol a release: Survey of the composition of dental composite resins. Open Dentistry Journal. 2016;**10**:446-453

[14] Li AJ, Kannan K. Elevated concentrations of bisphenols, benzophenones, and antimicrobials in pantyhose collected from six countries. Environmental Science & Technology. 2018;**52**:10812-10819

[15] Freire C, Molina-Molina JMJ-M, Iribarne-Duran LM, et al. Concentrations of bisphenol A and parabens in socks for infants and young children in Spain and their hormone-like

activities. Environment International. 2019;**127**:592-600

[16] Bacle A, Thevenot S, Grignon C, et al. Determination of bisphenol A in water and the medical devices used in hemodialysis treatment. International Journal of Pharmaceutics. 2016;**505**:115-121

[17] ASTM International. ASTM D7611/D7611M - 18 Standard practice for coding plastic manufactured articles for resin identification. Available from: https://www.astm.org/Standards/D7611.htm [Accessed: January 5, 2018]

[18] ASTM International. ASTM plastics committee releases major revisions to resin identification code (RIC) standard. Available from: https://www.astm.org/cms/drupal-7.51/newsroom/astm-plastics-committee-releases-major-revisions-resin-identification-code-ric-standard [Accessed: January 5, 2018]

[19] D20.95 Jurisdiction Page. Subcommittee D20.95 on Recycled Plastics. Matching Standards Under the Jurisdiction of D20.95 by Status. Available from: https://www.astm.org/jurisdiction-d2095 [Accessed: November 10, 2022]

[20] Konieczna A, Rutkowska A, Rachon D, et al. Health risk of exposure to bisphenol A (BPA). Roczniki Państwowego Zakładu Higieny. 2015;**66**:5-11

[21] Pérez W. Conozca lo que alerta el triángulo en los envases de plástico. la Razón. 2018

[22] Merino R. Qué botellas de plástico se pueden rellenar y cuáles son las alternativas?. Diario Sur. 2019

[23] Viciosa M. Tiques, táperes y biberones: Riesgos y mitos del bisfenol A. El Independiente. 2019

[24] Cao X-L, Popovic S. Solid phase extraction of large volume of water and beverage samples to improve detection limits for GC-MS analysis of bisphenol A and four other bisphenols. Food Additives & Contaminants. Part A, Chemistry, Analysis, Control, Exposure & Risk Assessment. 2018;**35**:49-55

[25] Wang H, Zhua L, Tang Z, et al. Bisphenol analogues in Chinese bottled water: Quantification and potential risk analysis. Science of the Total Environment. 2020;**713**:136583

[26] Guart A, Bono-Blay F, Borrell A, et al. Migration of plasticizersphthalates, bisphenol A and alkylphenols from plastic containers and evaluation of risk. Food Additives & Contaminants. Part A, Chemistry, Analysis, Control, Exposure & Risk Assessment. 2011;**28**:676-685

[27] Hermabessiere L, Dehaut A, Paul-Pont I, et al. Occurrence and effects of plastic additives on marine environments and organisms: A review. Chemosphere. 2017;**182**:781-793

[28] Suhrhoff TJ, Scholz-Böttcher BM. Qualitative impact of salinity, UV radiation and turbulence on leaching of organic plastic additives from four common plastics - A lab experiment. Marine Pollution Bulletin. 2016;**102**:84-94

[29] Simoneau C, Van den Eede L, Valzacchi S. Identification and quantification of the migration of chemicals from plastic baby bottles used as substitutes for polycarbonate. Food Additives & Contaminants. Part A, Chemistry, Analysis, Control, Exposure & Risk Assessment. 2012;**29**:469-480

[30] Moreno-Gómez-Toledano R, Arenas MI, Sánchez-Esteban S, et al. Critical Analysis of Human Exposure to Bisphenol a and its Novel Implications on

Renal, Cardiovascular and Hypertensive Diseases. In: Heshmati HM, editor. Hot Topics in Endocrinology and Metabolism. London, UK: IntechOpen; 2021. pp. 1-20

[31] Rochester JR, Bolden AL. Bisphenol S and F: A systematic review and comparison of the hormonal activity of bisphenol a substitutes. Environmental Health Perspectives. 2015;**123**:643-650

[32] Liu B, Lehmler HJ, Sun Y, et al. Association of Bisphenol A and Its Substitutes, Bisphenol F and Bisphenol S, with Obesity in United States Children and Adolescents. Diabetes and Metabolism Journal. 2019;**43**:59-75

[33] Mendy A, Salo PMPM, Wilkerson J, et al. Association of urinary levels of bisphenols F and S used as bisphenol A substitutes with asthma and hay fever outcomes. Environmental Research. 2020;**183**:108944

[34] Wang Y, Aimuzi R, Nian M, et al. Bisphenol A substitutes and sex hormones in children and adolescents. Chemosphere. 2021;**278**:130396

[35] Bornehag CG, Engdahl E, Hallerback MU, et al. Prenatal exposure to bisphenols and cognitive function in children at 7 years of age in the Swedish SELMA study. Environment International. 2021;**150**:106433

[36] Jiang YQ, Li JF, Xu SQ, et al. Prenatal exposure to bisphenol A and its alternatives and child neurodevelopment at 2 years. Journal of Hazardous Materials. 2020;**388**:121774

[37] Kim JI, Lee YA, Shin CH, et al. Association of bisphenol A, bisphenol F, and bisphenol S with ADHD symptoms in children. Environment International. 2022;**161**:107093

Chapter 2

The "Plastic Age": From Endocrine Disruptors to Microplastics – An Emerging Threat to Pollinators

Rafael Moreno-Gómez-Toledano and Clara Jabal-Uriel

Abstract

Currently, human beings live in a new era, known as the "Plastic Age." Throughout the history of plastics, two significant potential hazards to human health have been identified. Firstly, the endocrine-disrupting capability of monomers used in plastic synthesis has been under scrutiny. Secondly, in recent years, the potential dangers of nano- and microplastics released from the polymers themselves have begun to gain visibility, with their abundance and health consequences still under study. Consequently, this chapter begins with an analysis of xenobiotic compounds and endocrine disruptors. Subsequently, this chapter emphasizes the concept of microplastics, as their limited number of publications contrasts with their ubiquitous global distribution and potential harmful effects. Their presence across terrestrial ecosystems raises concerns about the possible impacts on pollinator health as these animals are crucial for maintaining agricultural production and plant biodiversity. The quantification of these particles in honey, beeswax, or the pollinators themselves could enable the assessment of the environmental impact of microplastics in terrestrial ecosystems, together with other pollutants that endanger these species. Nevertheless, more research is needed to evaluate the potential threat of microplastics and potential synergies among microplastics and other pollutants found in nature as a consequence of anthropogenic activities.

Keywords: plastic age, endocrine disruptors, microplastics, pollinators, honeybees

1. Introduction

Contemporary society exists in a distinct historical period, often referred to by some authors as the "Plastic Age". This nomenclature stems from the ever-expanding influence of plastics, which are now imprinting a lasting mark on terrestrial and aquatic environments across the globe [1, 2]. In the present day, plastics have become a common feature in a wide range of everyday items, owing to the heavy dependence of various industries on plastic polymers. Plastics have become an integral part of our lives, influencing how products are packaged, transported, and utilized, while also driving technological advancements. The underlying issue is that their production, use, disposal, and recycling involve the release of various particles that have never been found in the natural environment or circulating in the population's bloodstream until now. From a quantitative perspective, more than 200 compounds, called xenobiotic compounds, have been identified that should not be present within any living organism [3]. These compounds can be defined as:

> *"Organic chemicals that are not products of biosynthesis" [4] or*
>
> *"A xenobiotic is a chemical which is not a natural component of the organism exposed to it. Synonyms: drug, foreign substance or compound, exogenous substance or compound" [5].*

In light of their enduring presence and extensive distribution, an increasing number of authors are focusing their attention on the potential link between environmental xenobiotics and the development of various physiological disturbances or pathologies, with particular emphasis on exploring the deleterious effects of endocrine disruptors [6–10]. The concept of endocrine disruptors is relatively recent. While the knowledge of synthetic compounds capable of mimicking hormonal actions dates back to the early twentieth century, exemplified by bisphenol A (BPA),[1] it was not until the 1990s that the term was officially coined. It was during this period that a heightened awareness emerged regarding the potential association between exposure to environmental contaminants and an elevated risk of developing pathologies. The initial definition proposed by a public body, the United States Environmental Protection Agency[2] (EPA), characterizes an endocrine disruptor as:

> *"An exogenous chemical substance or mixture that alters the structure or function(s) of the endocrine system and causes adverse effects at the level of the organism, its progeny, populations, or subpopulations of organisms, based on scientific principles, data, weight-of-evidence, and the precautionary principle" [13].*

Subsequently, successive definitions have been proposed by the European Union and the US Environmental Protection Agency [12, 14], or various institutions, such as the World Health Organization [15]. However, for The Endocrine Society,[3] these definitions are problematic when placed in the context of hazard and risk characterization. Only one of them, the one made by the EPA (detailed in the previous paragraph), better fits the concept of endocrine disruptor as an external element influenced by environmental chemicals, capable of affecting the endocrine system in some way. Therefore, they propose a definition within the theoretical line of the EPA, but using simpler language:

---

[1] This phenolic-type monomer presents an intriguing dichotomy as it is one of the most widely used due to its remarkable versatility (serving as a monomer, additive, and plasticizer [11]), while simultaneously being one of the most extensively studied for its potential to function as a hormone, effectively acting as an endocrine disruptor [12].

[2] The definition comes specifically from the report made by the federal advisory committee, called the Endocrine Disruptor Screening and Testing Advisory Committee (EDSTAC), charged with making recommendations to the EPA. It was created following the passage of the Food Quality Protection Act (FQPA) in August 1996 [13].

[3] "Founded in 1916, The Endocrine Society is the world's oldest, largest, and most active organization devoted to research on hormones and the clinical practice of endocrinology" [12].

> *"An ED is an exogenous chemical, or mixture of chemicals, that interferes with any aspect of hormone action" [12].*

Currently, one of the most interesting and complete definitions of the concept can be found in Dr. Nicolás Olea's book "Libérate de tóxicos" (Free yourself from toxics), which states:

> *"Endocrine disruptors are chemical substances capable of altering the synthesis, release, transport, metabolism, binding, action or elimination of natural hormones in the organism, i.e., with the ability to alter hormonal balance and the regulation of embryonic development and, therefore, with the potential to cause adverse effects on the health of an organism or its offspring." (Translated from [16]).*

Within the broad diversity of molecules that make up this new group of xenobiotics compounds, However, there is a changing trend in the study of plastics, since in recent years it has been observed that not only low molecular weight monomers can have an impact on human health, but that abrasive action on any plastic element could contribute to its disintegration, creating countless nano and micro scale particles [17].

2. Microplastics

The concept of "microplastics" (MPs) still lacks a universal definition, although it is common in the literature to define them as any plastic particles with a size smaller than 5 mm. When it comes to particles smaller than 1 µm in size, the term "nanoplastics" is often used [18, 19]. Hence, we can come across various nomenclatures used to define the same concept. Leslie et al. [18] employ the term "plastic particles" to avoid ambiguity, while Sripada et al. [20] use the term "nano- and microplastics (NMPs)."

These types of particles fall into the category of "contaminants of emerging concern" because they have been detected in the environment, may have an impact on ecosystems or human health, and are not yet regulated by environmental laws [21]. Microplastics have been identified in numerous settings, locations, and matrices. From the water, food, and air in our immediate surroundings to remote environments like mountains and seas, microplastics have become unwelcome guests in our lives [18, 21].

The most obvious consequence of the ubiquity of microplastics is human exposure, which is a clear reality as their presence has been detected in urine [22], feces [23], and even in human blood and placenta [18, 24].

However, the major issue concerning microplastics is the determination of the true extent of the problem, that is, the ability to realistically quantify microplastic pollution in the environment and, consequently, the potential danger that numerous animal and plant species, as well as humans, are facing.

3. Microplastics in terrestrial ecosystems

The first studies assessing the presence of MPs particles in natural environments have focused mainly in aquatic ecosystems and marine biota, which have received attention since these particles have been found in oceanic and coastal locations across the globe [25–27] as well as in freshwater [28]. Even though many studies have focused on the potential harm of MPs in aquatic ecosystems, studies on the effects of these particles in terrestrial ecosystems are increasing [29, 30]. Considering that most of the plastic waste originates on land as a result of anthropic activities [31, 32], it is logic to consider that MPs produce alterations and interact with species in these ecosystems as well. In fact, MPs can accumulate in soil, altering its biophysical environment [29, 33] and ultimately entering in the food chain.

Recent evidence is extremely concerning, as there are studies like Shan et al. [34], in which they have observed the ability of polystyrene nanoplastics to cross the blood-brain barrier and induce neurotoxicity in a mouse model study. Similarly, Jin et al. [35] administered polystyrene microplastics (PS-MPs) in drinking water to mice and observed the accumulation of these particles in the brains of the treated animals. Their findings suggested that PS-MPs could disrupt the blood-brain barrier, impair learning and memory, and induce neurotoxicity in mice. However, more research needs to be done on how results obtained from experiments translate to the concentrations found in nature [33].

Moreover, most studies have focused on how these compounds have an effect in humans and other mammals, while disregarding numerous wild species. In this sense, insects are the widest group of the animal kingdom and form the base of the trophic chain within terrestrial ecosystems. One of the services they provide to the environment, along with other species, is pollination. The omnipresence of MPs facilitates that pollinators contact these particles that adhere to their bodies while feeding on flowers on enter their bodies by drinking freshwater.

4. Importance of pollinators

Pollinators are key pieces of terrestrial ecosystems and underpin its successful functioning [36, 37]. A large number of plant species depend on these animals to fertilize and reproduce, and have co-evolved since ancient times [38], and these relationships are essential to maintain the ecological communities [39, 40]. Pollination can occur *via* wind or water, and *via* animal [38]. Although the abiotic factors are used by some species, it is estimated that nearly 90% of plants worldwide need animal pollination [41]. The communication between pollinators and plants is mutually beneficial, since pollinators feed on nectar and pollen, floral rewards, while enhance plant's reproductive success by transporting pollen among flowers.

Pollination is crucial for agriculture, and in many countries, the use of insects is a common practice [42, 43]. Approximately, three quarters of agricultural production rely at least to some extent upon insect pollination [39, 44], and its worth is estimated in 235–577$ billion globally per year in crop and orchard pollination [44]. However, besides the economic value translated into food production, it is worth emphasizing the help in maintaining biodiversity.

On the one hand, honeybees (*Apis* spp.) and bumblebees (*Bombus* spp.) are the preferred and more widespread species used for pollination, although there are slight variations among continents [37]. Their adaptability and easy management make them very accessible to use. Moreover, in case of the honeybee, being a eusocial insect implies there might be thousands of individuals in a colony, which also facilitates their study, and it also provides hive products such as honey and wax, destined to human consumption. On the other hand, these two species are not the only ones found in the ecosystem. There are over 20,000 species of bees worldwide [43] and bees are not the only pollinators. Wild pollinators also comprise wild bees, flies, butterflies, beetles, wasps, moths and other insects as well as birds, bats and lizards. Wild pollinators have developed efficient pollinating systems and are of great importance since they pollinate crops more effectively [45].

5. Onset of research

The presence of NMPs in the terrestrial environment has become a huge concern for the scientific community and the general public. In these past years, the first studies have begun to analyze how the presence of these particles might influence pollinator health since one major outcome of the situation could be the disruption of plant-pollinator communication and the implications on biodiversity and food production. Many of the studies have been carried out in honeybees [46–49] and it could be expected that similar effects occur in other insect pollinating species. MPs have been found in apiaries in China [49] and honeybees have been used as samplers for microplastics in Denmark in urban and suburban areas [50]. However, experiments on the effects of MPs are usually carried out under laboratory conditions with short-term exposure [51], and pollinators exhibit varying responses to different sizes and concentrations of NMPs [30, 52].

6. Problems with NMPs in pollinators

Problems with NMPs in pollinators have been mainly recorded in honey bees due to the benefits of studying this species, mentioned above. Moreover, research has been carried out primarily in the laboratory, where ingestion of MPs has shown to sometimes alter the size [49], the gut microbiota [46], and the susceptibility to viral infections [49].

Although behavioral changes have been observed in aquatic animals after MPs ingestion, studies carried out in honeybees are scarce and have shown somewhat discrepant results. Buteler et al. [53] did not detect behavioral changes after MPs ingestion whereas Balzani et al. [48] found changes in feeding behavior depending on the administered MPs-concentration.

Laboratory studies have found that exposure to MPs of 0.1 μm significantly decreased body weight of honeybees [54] and MPs particles of 0.5 and 5 μm induced hair fall and changes in body color of adult honeybees [49] as opposed to bigger particles. MPs accumulated in the digestive tract might produce intestinal dysplasia [54] and also enter to other body parts such as the Malphigian tubules and the trachea, possibly through breakdown of the peritrophic membrane of the midgut [49] and transported within the hemolypmph. This is of great concern since honeybee gut microbiota might interact with MPs accumulated in the distal part of the digestive tract, the hindgut [54], whereas breakdown of the peritrophic membrane might cause impairment of the intestinal barrier functions and accentuate susceptibility of viral infection. Gut microbiota in honeybees is important to maintain its health and it is involved in nutrition processes [55], growth [56], immunity [57] and protection against pathogens [58], as gut microbiota has been studied to have similar roles in other insects. Honeybees fed with MPs decreased alpha diversity of gut microbiota [46] and it could have negative effects on their physiology. At individual level under laboratory conditions, MP consumption seems to compromise the immunity response and to alter gene expression [46], suggesting a reduced capacity for detoxification of xenobiotics and other pathogens [49].

Besides the effects that MPs have on honeybees, it is important to note that particles are ubiquitous in nature and can be found in their bodies, attached in their cuticles or in the digestive tracts [50, 53] and in other matrices of the hive [47], dispersing them to all the colony. MPs are found in contaminated water and food, and it has been suggested that the gear of beekeepers is another contamination source. MPs are incorporated from the environment by adult workers when foraging and these particles can be found in larvae, probably through nursing and feeding the larvae. More research needs to be done in order to evaluate possible consequences. Another possibility that has been observed in mosquitoes is that larvae ingested MPs and these particles remained in their adult stage after metamorphosis [59]. Once ingested by the honeybees, MPs are incorporated to the hive and stored mainly in the wax, probably because of the hydrophobic properties of plastic [47]. MPs can also be found in honey. Alma et al. found no significant differences in the MPs concentration in honey from their experimental hives and commercial honey, suggesting there is no contamination from MPs stored in wax to honey. At the end of their experiment, they did not find differences in honey reserves and bee population between the treated and the untreated group neither. As particles are ubiquitous and honey bees shared floral resources with other pollinating insects, it would be expected that these species also had attached particles in their bodies that were carried and stored in their nests, posing similar threats.

Mortality in honeybees fed with MPs was not significantly higher than in control groups [46, 53] and might appear that MPs are not the most toxic pollutant. Nevertheless, sub lethal effects must be considered, since they might affect pollinator's performance and fitness and have an impact on the immune response of honeybees. And it is a reason why mortality should be not used as an end point on colony performance. In this regard, López-Uribe et al. [60] proposed the term "pollinator health". It was defined as "a state that allows individuals to live longer and/or reproduce more (...) thus providing more ecological services", concept that uses other indicators and aspects of individual and colony performance of honeybees and other pollinators.

7. Other pollutants

MPs are able to adhere and to carry other xenobiotic compounds such as chemicals and pesticides, which increase the toxicity of MPs and mortality of pollinators [61]. Because of it, chemical effects could be greater than physical effects. For example, the use of the antibiotic tetracycline increased lethality in honeybees fed with MPs [46]. MPs are able to transport opportunistic bacteria that could harm the honeybee gut microbiota. In fact, the term "plastisphere" encompasses the microbial communities in plastic debris [62], and highlights the formation of ecosystems evolved to live in plastic environments. Besides bacteria and other microorganisms, MPs can adsorb other pollutants. Moreover, laboratory experiments tend to use spherical MPs particles whereas fibers have been also found in the field [49, 50]. Because fibers and other irregular shapes are more common in the environment, it is unclear how the concentrations, sizes and shapes used in experiments are representative in nature.

8. Considerations and future research perspectives

Honeybees have been traditionally used as a sentinel insect to monitor environmental quality [63], and they can be used to trace other contamination in the environment, not only MPs. Moreover, other matrices of the hive, such as pollen and propolis, can be analyzed for contamination of pesticides and other compounds.

Nevertheless, future research must evaluate how plastic pollution impacts on wild species of insects, given that biology, ecology, and genetics are important on the effect of contaminants as well as influence the routes of transmission and levels of exposure. For example, population of solitary insects might be more susceptible than social species, that is honeybees, where the loss of individuals does not pose such a threat to population and can cope better with the toxic compounds of the environment. Furthermore, research needs to focus on potential interactions between MPs and other compounds in field conditions, to better understand how they impact on honeybee and pollinator health. These future studies in field conditions should last longer in order to determine if contamination within hives has any impact on chronic health [47].

The problematic with MPs is difficult to solve, due to the dispersion of pollutants across political borders. For this reason, a global framework must be established that allow countries to collaborate. However, until now environmental regulations are quite permissive about MPs levels of industrial plants [30]. Studies with realistic concentrations of MPs close to those present in the environment are necessary in order to estimate health risks in the environment and in pollinators. Apart from this, it is necessary to use standardized protocols and report results in the same concentration units, since the use of different MPs composition and sizes and shapes across studies makes it difficult to compare them [47].

Extra effort should be implementing of pollinator conservation policies due to their decline could lead to impairment in plant-pollinator biology. This problem has many layers, since pollinators are not only affected by MPs. A holistic and interdisciplinary approach needs to be adopted to deal with the situations that are putting on edge the conservation of pollinators.

9. Final statement

Modern society is confronted with new challenges and issues related to everyday products, which often contain an abundance of plastic polymers in their structure. Despite the limited number of academic publications exploring the potential deleterious effects of NMPs, the experience of recent decades with endocrine disruptors and the current body of evidence should be sufficient to prompt authorities and governments to act. While an outright ban on plastics may be economically challenging in the current context, it is essential to implement actions aimed at environmental health literacy. Associations, institutions, and governments must promote awareness campaigns regarding the ecological impact of plastics and their effects on public health. Additionally, governments should take into consideration the precautionary principle considering current scientific evidence and promote measures to limit the use of plastics, particularly in the context of food.

As a result, environmental health literacy should bring attention to the plastic issue and promote small actions that gradually resonate within society. The goal is to progressively modify people's lifestyles, leading them toward more sustainable ways of living with reduced plastic usage. Because of the ever-evolving political environment, it is typical for policies and changes to be put into action on a short-term basis. In this sense, the World Health Organization developed the One Health Initiative, an approach that aims to balance and optimize the health of people, animals, and the environment as a whole. In this context, governments, stakeholders, and researchers should work together to manage health threats such as the ones mentioned in this chapter. It is essential to acknowledge that the necessary changes in this case have far-reaching implications for the fabric of society and should be cultivated over the course of generations. The actions we take today will impact the future of humanity.

Acknowledgements

The authors want to thank Elisa Moreno-Mizileanu for her indispensable logistical support.

Conflict of interest

The authors declare no conflict of interest.

Author details

Rafael Moreno-Gómez-Toledano[1*] and Clara Jabal-Uriel[2*]

1 Department of Surgery, Medical and Social Sciences, Area of Human Anatomy and Embryology, Universidad de Alcalá, Alcalá de Henares, Spain

2 Laboratorio de Patología Apícola, Centro de Investigación Apícola y Agroambiental (CIAPA), Instituto Regional de Investigación y Desarrollo Agroalimentario y Forestal (IRIAF), Consejería de Agricultura de la Junta de Comunidades de Castilla-La Mancha, Marchamalo, Spain

*Address all correspondence to: rafael.moreno@uah.es and c.jabaluriel@outlook.es

References

[1] Porta R. Anthropocene, the plastic age and future perspectives. FEBS Open Bio. 2021;**11**:948-953

[2] Li Y, Zhang Q, Baartman J, et al. The plastic age: River pollution in China from crop production and urbanization. Environmental Science & Technology. 2023;**57**:12019-12032

[3] Buser MC, Ingber SZ. Fourth Report on Human Exposure to Environmental Chemicals, Updated Tables. Atlanta, GA: U. S. Department of Health and Human Services: Centers for Disease Control and Prevention; 2017

[4] Baveye P, Bladon R. Bioavailability of organic xenobiotics in the environment. A critical perspective. In: Baveye P, Jean-Claude B, Goncharuk VV, editors. Bioavailability of Organic Xenobiotics in the Environment. Dordrecht: Springer Netherlands; 1999. p. 504

[5] Mervyn R. Environmental Xenobiotics. Great Britain: Taylor & Francis; 1996. p. 453

[6] Fucic A, Gamulin M, Ferencic Z, et al. Environmental exposure to xenoestrogens and oestrogen related cancers: Reproductive system, breast, lung, kidney, pancreas, and brain. Environmental Health. 2012;**11**:S8

[7] Heindel JJ, Blumberg B, Cave M, et al. Metabolism disrupting chemicals and metabolic disorders. Reproductive Toxicology. 2017;**68**:3-33

[8] Petrakis D, Vassilopoulou L, Mamoulakis C, et al. Endocrine disruptors leading to obesity and related diseases. International Journal of Environmental Research and Public Health. 2017;**14**:1-18

[9] Foulds CE, Treviño LS, York B, et al. Endocrine-disrupting chemicals and fatty liver disease. Nature Reviews. Endocrinology. 2017;**13**:445-457

[10] Lang IA, Galloway TS, Scarlett A, et al. Association of urinary bisphenol a concentration with medical disorders and laboratory abnormalities in adults. JAMA. 2008;**300**:1303-1310

[11] Thomas S, Visakh P, editors. Handbook of Engineering and Specialty Thermoplastics, Polyethers and Polyesters. Vol. 3. Hoboken, NJ, USA: Wiley-Scrivener; 2011

[12] Zoeller RT, Brown TR, Doan LL, et al. Endocrine-disrupting chemicals and public health protection: A statement of principles from the Endocrine Society. Endocrinology. 2012;**153**:4097-4110

[13] Endocrine Disruptor Screening and Testing Advisory Committee. EDSTAC Final Report. 1998. Available from: https://www.epa.gov/sites/production/files/2015-08/documents/exesum14.pdf

[14] European Commission. COM(2018)734. Communication from the Commission to the European Parliament, the Council, the European Economic and Social Committee and the Committee of the Regions. Towards a Comprehensive European Union Framework on Endocrine Disruptors. 2018. Available from: https://ec.europa.eu/transparency/regdoc/rep/1/2018/ES/COM-2018-734-F1-ES-MAIN-PART-1.PDF [Accessed: 1 April 2023]

[15] Bergman Å, Heindel JJ, Jobling S, et al. State of the Science of Endocrine Disrupting Chemicals 2012. Geneva, Switzerland; 2013

[16] Olea N. Libérate de tóxicos. Guía para evitar los disruptores endocrinos. 1st ed. Barcelona, España: RBA Libros S.A; 2019

[17] Blöcker L, Watson C, Wichern F. Living in the plastic age - different short-term microbial response to microplastics addition to arable soils with contrasting soil organic matter content and farm management legacy. Environmental Pollution. 2020;**267**:115468

[18] Leslie HA, van Velzen MJM, Brandsma SH, et al. Discovery and quantification of plastic particle pollution in human blood. Environment International. 2022;**163**:107199

[19] Dick Vethaak A, Legler J. Microplastics and human health. Science. 2021;**371**:672-674

[20] Sripada K, Wierzbicka A, Abass K, et al. A children's health perspective on nano- and microplastics. Environmental Health Perspectives. 2022;**130**(1):15001

[21] Mitrano DM, Wick P, Nowack B. Placing nanoplastics in the context of global plastic pollution. Nature Nanotechnology. 2021;**16**:491-500

[22] Pironti C, Notarstefano V, Ricciardi M, et al. First evidence of microplastics in human urine, a preliminary study of intake in the human body. Toxics. 2022;**11**(1):40

[23] Zhang N, Bin LY, He HR, et al. You are what you eat: Microplastics in the feces of young men living in Beijing. Science of the Total Environment. 2021;**767**:144345

[24] Ragusa A, Svelato A, Santacroce C, et al. Plasticenta: First evidence of microplastics in human placenta. Environment International. 2021;**146**:106274

[25] Carvalho Ferreira H, Lôbo-Hajdu G. Microplastics in coastal and oceanic surface waters and their role as carriers of pollutants of emerging concern in marine organisms. Marine Environmental Research. 2023;**188**:10621

[26] Huang L, Zhang S, Li L, et al. Research progress on microplastics pollution in polar oceans. Polar Science. 2023;**36**:100946

[27] Khoshmanesh M, Sanati AM, Ramavandi B. Co-occurrence of microplastics and organic/inorganic contaminants in organisms living in aquatic ecosystems: A review. Marine Pollution Bulletin. 2023;**187**:114563

[28] Khan ML, Hassan HU, Khan FU, et al. Effects of microplastics in freshwater fishes health and the implications for human health. Brazilian Journal of Biology. 2024;**84**:1-16

[29] Sun Y, Duan C, Cao N, et al. Effects of microplastics on soil microbiome: The impacts of polymer type, shape, and concentration. Science of the Total Environment. 2022;**806**:150516

[30] de Souza Machado AA, Kloas W, Zarfl C, et al. Microplastics as an emerging threat to terrestrial ecosystems. Global Change Biology. 2018;**24**:1405-1416

[31] Li W, Zu B, Yang Q, et al. Sources, distribution, and environmental effects of microplastics: A systematic review. RSC Advances. 2023;**13**:15566-15574

[32] Osman AI, Hosny M, Eltaweil AS, et al. Microplastic sources, formation, toxicity and remediation: A review. Environmental Chemistry Letters. 2023;**4**:1-41

[33] Wang W, Ge J, Yu X, et al. Environmental fate and impacts of microplastics in soil ecosystems: Progress and perspective. Science of the Total Environment. 2020;**708**:134841

[34] Shan S, Zhang Y, Zhao H, et al. Polystyrene nanoplastics penetrate across the blood-brain barrier and induce activation of microglia in the brain of mice. Chemosphere. 2022;**298**:134261

[35] Jin H, Yang C, Jiang C, et al. Evaluation of neurotoxicity in BALB/c mice following chronic exposure to polystyrene microplastics. Environmental Health Perspectives. 2022;**130**(10):107002

[36] Gill RJ, Baldock KCR, Brown MJF, et al. Protecting an ecosystem service: Approaches to understanding and mitigating threats to wild insect pollinators. Advances in Ecological Research. 2016;**54**:135-206

[37] Brondizio ES, Settele J, Díaz S, Ngo HT, editors. IPBES: Global Assessment Report on Biodiversity and Ecosystem Services of the Intergovernmental Science-Policy Platform on Biodiversity and Ecosystem Services. Bonn, Germany: IPBES Secretariat; 2019. p. 1148

[38] Fattorini R, Glover BJ. Molecular mechanisms of pollination biology. Annual Review of Plant Biology. 2020;**71**:487-515

[39] Klein AM, Vaissière BE, Cane JH, et al. Importance of pollinators in changing landscapes for world crops. Proceedings of the Royal Society B: Biological Sciences. 2007;**274**:303-313

[40] Bishop J, Garratt MPD, Nakagawa S. Animal pollination increases stability of crop yield across spatial scales. Ecology Letters. 2022;**25**:2034-2047

[41] Ollerton J. Pollinator diversity: Distribution, ecological function, and conservation. Annual Review of Ecology, Evolution, and Systematics. 2017;**48**:353-376

[42] vanEngelsdorp D, Meixner MD. A historical review of managed honey bee populations in Europe and the United States and the factors that may affect them. Journal of Invertebrate Pathology. 2010;**103**:S80-S95

[43] European Commission, Directorate-General for Environment. Pollinators – Importance for Nature and Human Well-being, Drivers of Decline and the Need for Monitoring. Publications Office; 2020

[44] Potts SG, Biesmeijer JC, Bommarco R, et al. Status and Trends of European Pollinators. Key Findings of the STEP Project. Pensoft Publishers; 2015

[45] Garibaldi LA, Steffan-dewenter I, Winfree R, et al. Wild pollinators enhance fruit set of crops regardless of honey bee abundance. Science. 2014;**339**:1608-1611

[46] Wang K, Li J, Zhao L, et al. Gut microbiota protects honey bees (*Apis mellifera* L.) against polystyrene microplastics exposure risks. Journal of Hazardous Materials. 2021;**402**:123828

[47] Alma AM, de Groot GS, Buteler M. Microplastics incorporated by honeybees from food are transferred to honey, wax and larvae. Environmental Pollution. 2023;**320**:121078

[48] Balzani P, Galeotti G, Scheggi S, et al. Acute and chronic ingestion of polyethylene (PE) microplastics has mild effects on honey bee health and cognition. Environmental Pollution. 2022;**305**:119318

[49] Deng Y, Jiang X, Zhao H, et al. Microplastic polystyrene ingestion promotes the susceptibility of honeybee to viral infection. Environmental Science and Technology. 2021;**55**:11680-11692

[50] Edo C, Fernández-Alba AR, Vejsnæs F, et al. Honeybees as active

samplers for microplastics. Science of the Total Environment. 2021;**767**:144481

[51] Baho DL, Bundschuh M, Futter MN. Microplastics in terrestrial ecosystems: Moving beyond the state of the art to minimize the risk of ecological surprise. Global Change Biology. 2021;**27**:3969-3986

[52] Muhammad A, Zhou X, He J, et al. Toxic effects of acute exposure to polystyrene microplastics and nanoplastics on the model insect, silkworm Bombyx mori. Environmental Pollution. 2021;**285**:117255

[53] Buteler M, Alma AM, Stadler T, et al. Acute toxicity of microplastic fibers to honeybees and effects on foraging behavior. Science of the Total Environment. 2022;**822**:153320

[54] Wang K, Zhu L, Rao L, et al. Nano- and micro-polystyrene plastics disturb gut microbiota and intestinal immune system in honeybee. Science of the Total Environment. 2022;**842**:156819

[55] Branchiccela B, Castelli L, Corona M, et al. Impact of nutritional stress on the honeybee colony health. Scientific Reports. 2019;**9**:10156

[56] Zheng H, Powell JE, Steele MI, et al. Honeybee gut microbiota promotes host weight gain via bacterial metabolism and hormonal signaling. Proceedings of the National Academy of Sciences of the United States of America. 2017;**114**:4775-4780

[57] Emery O, Schmidt K, Engel P. Immune system stimulation by the gut symbiont Frischella perrara in the honey bee (*Apis mellifera*). Molecular Ecology. 2017;**26**:2576-2590

[58] Steele MI, Motta EVS, Gattu T, et al. The gut microbiota protects bees from invasion by a bacterial pathogen. Microbiology Spectrum. 2021;**9**(2):e0039421

[59] Al-Jaibachi R, Cuthbert RN, Callaghan A. Examining effects of ontogenic microplastic transference on Culex mosquito mortality and adult weight. Science of the Total Environment. 2019;**651**:871-876

[60] López-Uribe MM, Jha S, Soro A. A trait-based approach to predict population genetic structure in bees. Molecular Ecology. 2019;**28**:1919-1929

[61] Li J, Zhang K, Zhang H. Adsorption of antibiotics on microplastics. Environmental Pollution. 2018;**237**:460-467

[62] Amaral-Zettler LA, Zettler ER, Mincer TJ. Ecology of the plastisphere. Nature Reviews Microbiology. 2020;**18**:139-151

[63] Al Naggar Y, Brinkmann M, Sayes CM, et al. Are honey bees at risk from microplastics? Toxics. 2021;**9**:1-8

Chapter 3

Using New Online Databases to Identify Environmental Justice Issues

Michael Greenberg, Henry Mayer, David Kosson and Timothy Fields

Abstract

During the last decade, U.S. government agencies have published multiple online geographical databases. Containing demographic, environmental, public health, and urban service information, they permit users to examine environmental justice issues at county, city, and census tract scales. After briefly describing the opportunities associated with these sources, we illustrate their use to inform government policy with examples drawn from the U.S. Department of Energy's environmental management program. These examples include ranking of site areas regarding their need for environmental-justice-related assistance and the identification of opportunities to work with local colleges. The illustrations highlight the strengths and limitations of these databases and suggest ideas for increasing their utility to researchers and the general public. We strongly believe that these databases will expand and become even more useful.

Keywords: new online public databases, environmental and social justice, U.S. Department of Energy, local colleges, environmental health

1. Introduction

This chapter has two objectives. The first is to summarize five major new publicly available databases released by the U.S. Environmental Protection Agency, the U.S. Centers for Disease Control and Prevention (CDC), the U.S. Council on Environmental Quality (CEQ), and the University of Wisconsin. These databases allow researchers and the public to examine a wide variety of demographic, environmental, and public health and service datasets at the census tract, local government, county, and state scales and compare results across scales. The second objective is to illustrate these tools with several current challenging opportunities faced by the U.S. Department of Energy (DOE).

2. Five databases

We begin by describing five databases that allow researchers and members of the public to gain a holistic view of communities in the United States.

The U.S. government and others have been collecting data about people and businesses and publishing summaries of these since 1790. However, the 1950 census is the first one that is accessible to people looking for detained granular data. For many decades, researchers, including the first author, had to go to libraries and sort through thick books of data. Obtaining the data required hand copying it and then punching it on special cards before feeding it into a computer for analysis. To say it was a chore to secure the data from the paper files is an understatement. The new databases have created a much more user-friendly world.

2.1 EPA-EJScreen

As part of its obligations under President Clinton's (1994) Environmental Justice Order 12898 [1, 2] in 2010, the U.S.EPA committed to developing a publicly accessible database that would allow people to see how their area compared to others and for scientists to screen areas for specific characteristics. First released in 2015, it has been updated, most recently in 2023. Users can find information such as proportion of people of color, low income, less than a high school education, unemployment, and the youngest and oldest population. EPA's data is driven by the assumption that these are the most vulnerable populations. Also, indicators of air quality, automobile traffic density, location of hazardous materials and waste sites, and other environmental indicators are available.

The key strength of this database is having a built-in GIS tool that allows the user to draw circles, triangles, rectangles, and other polygons around a user-selected centroid. Hence, if the user does not choose to use census tracts, cities, or counties, s/he can explore other data collection shapes, which is critical because it allows comparison of places of equal size and shape. The tool comes with a technical manual [2]. However, many people do not have the patience to read all of EPA's caveats about the data. For example, the air pollution data are only as good as the density of monitors, which are limited in places. Also, even though the number of hazardous waste, storage tanks, and other data are calculated, their presence does not mean that anyone is being exposed. The 2022 update added important information such as broadband access, unemployment, climate change, and medically underserved populations.

2.2 CDC-PLACES

Supported by the Robert Wood Johnson Foundation, PLACES is a CDC database organized around census tracts to help local health officials [3]. In its early days, PLACES focused only on the 500 most populated cities in the United States. Users could obtain data but also were able to view mapped census tract data for the period 2016–2019. Twenty-seven metrics are available mostly for outcomes and prevention, with a few for health risk behaviors and self-assessed health status. The database was expanded in 2020 to provide small area estimates for all counties, incorporated jurisdictions, census tracts, and ZIP codes in the United States. Users can download data as well as view data on an interactive map. Like the EJScreen data, the challenge is to find your way through the various screens and, most importantly, to understand what the data is telling you. This is a powerful set of tools to mix with the data in EJScreen. There will be a learning curve for those not familiar with public health methods, such as age adjustment.

DOI: http://dx.doi.org/10.5772/intechopen.1001931

2.3 CEQ-CEJST

In early 2022, the Council on Environmental Quality (CEQ) [4] released an initial version of its Climate and Economic Justice Screening Tool (CEJST) that was developed to provide a uniform definition of disadvantaged communities for federal agencies to use in targeting their allocations under President Biden's Justice40 covered programs in the areas of climate, clean energy and energy efficiency, clean transit, affordable and sustainable housing, training and workforce development, the remediation and reduction of legacy pollution, and the development of clean water infrastructure. The tool uses datasets and methodologies to identify communities that are economically disadvantaged and overburdened by pollution and underinvestment in housing, transportation, water and wastewater infrastructure, and health care. CEJST relies on income, education, environmental burdens, health, and other economic and environmental factors at the census tract level. The user can compare the percent of the population in each tract relative to a nationally measured metric for each indicator. A community, as represented by a census tract, is deemed by the CEJST to be "disadvantaged" if (i) it is above the CEQ established threshold for one or more environmental or climate indicators and (ii) it is also above the threshold for all of the socioeconomic indicators. The tract must satisfy both criteria to be considered disadvantaged.

CEQ's approach elicited hundreds of suggestions, including from these authors [5]. When CEQ revised their approach, many of the objections were addressed. The advantage of the CEQ's approach is users can look directly at census tract data, which is close to a neighborhood of 4000–8000 people in most cases. The main disadvantage is that a census tract can be declared eligible for assistance by crossing one disadvantaged category. In the U.S., this means that about one-third of the U.S.'s 84,000+ census tracts are "disadvantaged." Realistically, there are insufficient resources to help all of these places, and we suggest using county and statistical tools to group these disadvantaged places (see below).

2.4 University of Wisconsin: County Health Rankings & Roadmaps

Supported by the Robert Wood Johnson Foundation, the University of Wisconsin Population Institute [6] through County Health Rankings & Roadmaps (CHR&R) provides public health-related data for almost every county in the United States. Users can secure county-scale data, guidance on how to use it through emails, webinars, and podcasts. Most importantly, the user can see the overlap between health behaviors, health outcomes, social indicators, and services.

For example, the first author lives in Middlesex County, NJ. In less than one minute, he found that Middlesex is ranked in the 50th–75th percentile in health outcomes in New Jersey as well as in health factors that influence health outcomes. The database has 14 health outcome measures and 60 health factors including behaviors, clinical care attributes of the area, socioeconomic factors, and physical environmental factors. Many of these are used to rank each county in the context of its host state and the United States. The data can be downloaded by year back to 2010. The only important limitation is that the data stops at the county scale, and it does not provide data at the municipal or census tract levels.

2.5 CDC, ATSDR, and The Department of Health and Human Services: Cumulative environmental justice

In August 2022, the Environmental Justice Index (EJI) [7] was released to capture what these several organizations consider the cumulative impacts of environmental burdens, that is, the total impact from a combination of environmental factors. The objective is to provide a single environmental justice score for local areas. The database contains 36 indicators divided into environmental burden, social vulnerability, and health vulnerability.

Cumulative impacts are the total harm to human health that occurs from the combination of environmental burden such as pollution and poor environmental conditions, preexisting health conditions, and social factors. It is the first national, geographic-driven tool designed to measure the cumulative impacts of environmental burden through the lenses of human health and health equity. The authors were briefed about this latest database and tested it with some sample data. However, we have not personally used it in for a major study. Hence, we have no insights based on in-depth work with the database.

3. Two case studies

3.1 Prioritizing places that need EJ program assistance: County scale

The U.S. federal government has a long history of helping distressed places and populations. The Marshall Plan and Japan after World War II are illustrative [8, 9]. Within the U.S., the Appalachia area has benefited from ongoing support [10], as well as federal Superfund and brownfield programs, and grants to help build sewage treatment facilities have made a major difference, and many others.

The Biden Administration created a federally funded Justice40 Initiative [11] that requires federal agencies to provide 40% of the benefits of their climate, clean energy, clean water, affordable and sustainable housing, and several other investments to disadvantaged communities that are marginalized, underserved, and stressed by pollution. The Department of Energy (DOE), indeed every federal agency, faces a challenging opportunity to meet this objective. DOE's environmental management program is addressing the large environmental legacy of its former nuclear weapons research and manufacturing operations. It is the single largest long-term federal program and its cost was estimated at over $500 in the year 2020 and growing [12]. DOE's funds are heavily concentrated at a few locations, unlike federal money for social security, Medicare, highways, and other programs that spread dollars across the country. Third, because of the huge cost, DOE sites are perceived as places to find budget reductions.

DOE's largest sites have been called "state-anchored regions" made dependent and left with a negative legacy [13]. Brauer [14, 15] asserted that DOE-centered regions had a bifurcated labor market and that private industry would not move to these areas because if DOE chose to create new missions the companies would not be able to match DOE's economic packages, and they would leave to work for DOE. Hooks and Getz [16] observed that from 1970 into the 1990s the large DOE-site regions were unique among federal agencies in not attracting private business to their regions. DOE's smaller Brookhaven (New York region), Rocky Flats (Denver), Fernald (Cincinnati), Argonne (Chicago), and Lawrence Livermore (San Jose and

San Francisco) sites are in or close to major metropolitan regions that can attract new activities to empty space. However, most of these sites have been closed. Savannah River, Idaho, Hanford, Portsmouth, and Paducah are not. While some have argued for economic assistance for these dependent regions, others asserted that steel mills, chemical plants, mines, and other private enterprise facilities had closed, and no such direct aid programs were created for them [17].

The DOE's large and ongoing operations in erstwhile rural regions represent one important piece of historical context; the second is the argument that DOE owes the large rural site areas additional support. The federal government purchased and/or confiscated large parcels of land at Savannah River, Oak Ridge, Hanford, and elsewhere that had been at least partly occupied. Residents were given a short time to leave. Some relocated outside the area, but others relocated nearby. Economist Milton Russell [18] made a case that the federal government should split allocations to these sites into operations and additional payments to account for the legacy. For example, Aiken (SC) and Benton's (WA) demographic profiles are different than its neighbors, partly shaped by DOE operations and by its pre-DOE history [19, 20]. In short, what is a reasonable amount of aid for places that were taken over by the federal government leaving long-term environmental and political legacies? In the case of DOE's large rural sites, federal investments in energy science and engineering, infrastructure, environmental justice, and climate change are pertinent to the ongoing DOE activity and historical legacies.

Given this legacy, we focus the illustrations on answering two questions:

1. Regarding economic, demographic, environmental, and health indicators, how much difference is there between the core counties hosting DOE's 10 major sites and the surrounding counties?

2. How can the data be used to prioritize the counties into having a need for EJ-related assistance?

Ten DOE sites accounted for over $6.5 billion (82%) of $7.9 billion allocated across the complex [21] for environmental cleanup. We focused on the 54 counties surrounding these DOE EM's sites having the most expensive legacy (**Table 1**). DOE will be at the sites for the foreseeable future. Accordingly, comparative studies are valuable for tracking the evolution of on-the-ground conditions in the surrounding regions that may influence the DOE's decisions. The geographical focus of this study are the ten counties that host these DOE site operations, the ten host counties adjacent to them, and the 34 adjacent to the host counties. The DOE core host counties (group 1) are small urban nodes with major operations offices. The DOE has brought high wages to these areas, and we assumed that the ten core host counties would have relatively high wages per employee. However, other characteristics should be associated with these core host functions. One of these is more people, higher density of activity, more traffic, and hence more air emissions. The other ten host DOE counties (group 2) are part of the DOE-site region, but they are not the places where large sums of federal resources are received before being reallocated. The group 3 counties are adjacent to the Group 1 and 2 counties and should be less directly impacted by DOE activities.

More than 100 metrics were available for this analysis. We picked six each to represent economic, environmental, public health, and demographic attributes. Eleven are from the EPA's EJScreen database, 10 from the University of Wisconsin's, two from the U.S. Census Bureau, and one from a private source. Please note that we

Site (n = number of counties)*	Core host county	Adjacent DOE host counties	Counties adjacent to host counties
Current DOE site region (n = 54)	**Group 1 10 inner host counties**	**Group 2 10 other host counties**	**Group 3 34 adjacent to host counties**
1a- Hanford Office of River Protection and 1-b Hanford Operations Office, WA (n = 5)	Benton	Franklin	Grant, Walla Walla, Yakima
2- Idaho National Laboratory, ID (n = 4)	Bonneville		Bingham, Jefferson, Madison
3- Los Alamos National Laboratory, NM (n = 8)	Los Alamos	Rio Arriba, Santa Fe, Taos	Colfax, Mora, Sandoval, Torrance
4- Moab, UT (n = 4)	Grand		Emery, San Juan, Uintah
5- Nevada National Security Site, NV (n = 4)	Nye		Esmerelda, Eureka, Lincoln
6-Oak Ridge, TN (n = 6)	Anderson	Roane	Cumberland, Knox, McMinn, Morgan
7- Paducah KY (n = 4)	McCracken		Ballard, Graves, Marshall
8-Portsmouth, OH (n = 7)	Pike	Jackson, Ross, Scioto	Gallia, Highland, Pickaway
9-Savannah River, SC (n = 8)	Aiken	Allendale, Barnwell	Bamberg, Edgefield, Hampton, Lexington, Orangeburg
10-WIPP, NM (n = 4)	Eddy		Chaves, Lea, Otero

*Source: [22].

Table 1.
Fifty-four counties included in the study.

make no assertion that these shed light on every issue related to the sites. Our goal was to pick representative metrics that are consistent with massive literature and available in federal databases. **Table 2** lists the 24 metrics used and summarizes the results.

The numbers in **Table 2**, with one exception, are standardized to host states, that is, test values of 100. For example, suppose state A's places had a median unemployment rate of 5%. Study area A5 had a value of 7.5%. By examining all the values in the state, we find that A5's value places it at the upper quartile in the state. The value in the table for area A5 would be 150 In other words, a value of 150 means that the site had a value 50% higher than the state's places, whereas a number of 50 means that that site has a much lower value than the host state's places. The numbers could theoretically range from 0 (lowest in the state) to 200 (highest in the state). We used one-way ANOVA tests and Tukey's-b post hoc test to measure statistical significance. However, given the small number of cases, the large size of the table, and to simplify the presentation, we present the 95% confidence limits for the numbers. The original reports present all the statistical significance tests [5, 23, 24].

The exception in the table is population change. Colleagues suggested that readers want to see the actual values. Hence, no change (0.0) is the test value.

The answers to question one are not subtle. The ten core host counties manifest stronger economic outcomes than the non-major host counties and the adjacent counties for all six indicators, better health outcomes for five of the six, and less

Metric	Major host counties, adjacent counties, and other sets of counties (n = 54)	Group Means*	(95 confidence limits)*
Economic (n = 6)			
Unemployment, 2019 (state test value =100)	Major host (n = 10) Non-major host (n = 10) Adjacent (n = 34)	112 133 116	(93,132) (110,156) (104,128)
Home value (state test value =100)	Major host (n = 10) Non-major host (n = 10) Adjacent (n = 34)	81 78 62	(64,98) (53,103) (55,70)
Severe housing cost challenge (state test value =100)	Major host (n = 10) Non-major host (n = 10) Adjacent (n = 34)	85 96 88	(69,102) (83,108) (76,100)
Broadband access (state test value =100)	Major host (n = 10) Non-major host (n = 10) Adjacent (n = 34)	100 89 92	(93,107) (81,97) (87,96)
Wages (test value =100) [values adjusted to median of each state's counties]	Major host (n = 10) Non-major host (n = 10) Adjacent (n = 34)	130 105 109	(109,150) (89,121) (100,118)
Population changes 2010–2020 (census counts) (test value =0)	Major host (n = 10) Non-major host (n = 10) Adjacent (n = 33)	3.4 −0.9 1.1	(0.5,6.4) (−5.9,4.1) (−1.3,3.5)
Environmental (n = 6)			
Pm 2.5 (state test value =100)	Major host (n = 10) Non-major host (n = 10) Adjacent (n = 34)	86 48 68	(30,142) (6,90) (46,90)
Ozone (state test value =100)	Major host (n = 10) Major adjacent (n = 10) Adjacent (n = 34)	78 50 64	(36,118) (10,90) (42,84)
Diesel particles (state test value =100)	Major host (n = 10) Non-major host (n = 10) Adjacent (n = 34)	54 42 44	(28,82) (14,70) (30,58)
Sites with chemical risk management plans (state test value =100)	Major host (n = 10) Non-major host (n = 10) Adjacent (n = 34)	98 96 94	(54,144) (56,136) (72,116)
Less than ½ mile from park (state test value =100)	Major host (n = 10) Non-major host (n = 10) Adjacent (n = 34)	92 58 75	(67,117) (34,83) (61,89)
Food environment (state test value =100)	Major host (n = 10) Non-major host (n = 10) Adjacent (n = 34)	118 119 113	(90,145) (97,141) (102,123)
Public Health (n = 6)			
Premature death rate (state test value =100)	Major host (n = 10) Non-major host (n = 10) Adjacent (n = 34)	117 114 115	(93,141) (79,149) (105,125)
Personal assessment of health as fair or poor, (state test value =100)	Major host (n = 10) Non-major host (n = 10) Adjacent (n = 34)	103 129 121	(87,119) (110,147) (114,128)
Adults lacking insurance (state test value =100)	Major host (n = 10) Non-major host (n = 10) Adjacent (n = 34)	94 103 107	(72,116) (77,129) (94,119)

Metric	Major host counties, adjacent counties, and other sets of counties (n = 54)	Group Means*	(95 confidence limits)*
Had flu shot, 2019 (state test value =100)	Major host (n = 10) Non-major host (n = 10) Adjacent (n = 34)	94 88 86	(72,116) (74,102) (80,93)
Covid-19 mortality rate, 2020 (state test value =100) Note only 93 counties had rates	Major host (n = 8) Non-major host (n = 10) Adjacent (n = 28)	99 110 120	(65,133) (67,154) (97,143)
Health factors, 2022 (test value =50, number in two best quartiles =1, others =0) Only 106 counties had rates	Major host (n = 10) Non-major host (n = 10) Adjacent (n = 33)	70 30 58	(35,105) (0,65) (40,75)
Demographic (n = 6)			
Low income, % (state test value =100)*	Major host (n = 10) Non-major host (n = 10) Adjacent (n = 34)	103 132 122	(78,134) (110,156) (112,134
Population of color, % (state test value =100)	Major host (n = 10) Non-major host (n = 10) Adjacent (n = 34)	82 112 94	(54,112) (76,148) (78,112)
Linguistic isolation, % (state test value =100)	Major host (n = 10) Non-major host (n = 10) Adjacent (n = 34)	124 130 132	(104,144) (114,146) (124,142)
Less than high school graduation, % (state test value =100)	Major host (n = 10) Non-major host (n = 10) Adjacent (n = 34)	112 134 126	(84,140) (110,160) (114,138)
Population < 5 years old, % (state test value =100)	Major host (n = 10) Non-major host (n = 10) Adjacent (n = 34)	102 100 100	(80,124) (80,122) (90,110)
Population > 64 years old, % (state test value =100)	Major host (n = 10) Non-major host (n = 10) Adjacent (n = 34)	130 124 124	(110,152) (100,148) (112,138)

**Numbers are rounded off to nearest whole number, with the exception of population change.*

Table 2.
Comparison of twenty-four metrics in fifty-four counties.

vulnerability for four of the six demographic measures. The exceptions are the premature death rate and the age groupings (>64 and < 5 years). The differences are small (5–25%) and not significantly different in post hoc tests because of small numbers of cases. Yet the consistency of these observations should not be ignored.

Regarding the environmental indicators, the inner core counties have poorer metrics regarding the three air pollutants and the presence of sites with risk management plans. Yet they have a better outcome for distance from parks. Overall, these results are consistent with the idea that the DOE's inner core counties have measurable benefits that are generally associated with an urban environment. Regarding environmental and social justice, these findings suggest that a good deal of resources are needed outside the host counties, indeed in some cases 100 miles away, which implies management and potentially political challenges.

We created a tool to score each of the 54 DOE counties and classify them into four "need" groups that approximate quartiles (Note that they are not quartiles because there are many ties). We used all 24 metrics in **Table 2**.

The simplest grouping was to assign each of the 24 variables an equal weight (4.168 out of 100 points). This is reported as the equal weight score (**Table 3**). We recognize that preferences vary. Accordingly, we created weighted cumulative scores around economics and demographics, which as noted earlier have been the two historic themes for the study areas. The weighting was done by valuing the economics metrics as being twice as important as any of the other metrics. In other words, the six economics metrics received 40 points, whereas the environment, public health, and demographic sets each received 20 points. The demographic weighted results weighted demographics as 40 points, and each of the three other sets were weighted 20 points. Also, we created a "rapid fix" score by focusing on five metrics: seasonal flu vaccination, obtaining health insurance, supporting those with severe housing cost needs, lack of broadband access, and lack of healthy food environment. These five could be addressed with short-term support but are not part of the historic DOE cleanup mission.

Table 3 lists the set of counties most and least in need. Hanford, Portsmouth, and Savannah River have nine of the ten most needy counties. Several observations are in order. One is that the groups do not change much with the weightings. The

Site & County (number of counties)	Equal weighting		Demographic weighting (40%)		Economic weighting (40%)		Rapid fix metrics	
	Number		Number		Number		Number	
	most needy	least needy	most needy	least needy	most needy	least needy	most needy	least needy
All ten sites (54)	10	13	12	13	12	12	9	20
Hanford (5)	3	0	4	0	3	0	1	0
Idaho National Laboratory (4)	0	1	0	1	0	1	0	2
Los Alamos National Laboratory (8)	0	3	0	3	0	3	0	5
Moab (4)	1	0	2	0	1	0	3	0
Nevada National Security Site (4)	0	2	0	2	0	2	1	0
Oak Ridge (6)	0	2	0	3	0	2	1	4
Paducah (4)	0	1	0	1	0	0	0	3
Portsmouth (7)	3	1	3	1	5	1	3	1
Savannah River (8)	3	1	3	1	3	1	0	2
Waste Isolation Pilot Plant (4)	0	2	0	1	0	2	0	3

Table 3.
Grouping of site areas into most and least in need groups.

correlations between the equally weighted scores and the demographic, economic, public health, and rapid fixes scores were r = 0.81, 0.69, 0.83, and 0.73, respectively (all significant at $P < 0.01$).

Clearly, need is clustered at three of the ten sites and within the sites tends to be in areas adjacent to the major site headquarters.

3.2 Upgrading educational programs

States, counties, cities, townships, and boroughs are the political units assigned to receive federal support. However, programs are typically implemented at neighborhood scales. In the United States, the census tracts are the closest units to neighborhoods. They are created by the U.S. Census Bureau and typically have 1200 to 8000 people. The United States has over 84,000 census tracts. The ten major DOE-EM sites have 770 census tracts in the 54 host counties. Data are available on more than 100 variables at the tract level from EPA, CEQ, US Census, CDC, and other reputable sources.

The empirical test that follows is a pilot restricted to eight counties and 150 census tracts that are around the Savannah River site (SRS). As the previous section shows, SRS had three of the ten counties most in need of assistance. The authors chose SRS because it is a large site (310 sq. mi./802.8 sq. km.) that is geographically surrounded by counties and communities with often markedly different socioeconomic and physical characteristics. Additionally, although active cleanup of the site provides employment and other economic benefits to these counties, SRS is also an active operating facility housing important DOE-Science and national security (NNSA) facilities. Thus, the site offers long-term economic opportunities and benefits to the surrounding region. Likewise, DOE will be reliant on these communities to provide an educated and trained workforce, specialized service business support, and overall political support for its continued presence in South Carolina.

In this illustration, we concentrate on improving educational achievement, but we also worked on efforts associated with expanding broadband access and assisting communities where many of their employees and families live in increasing the resilience of their vulnerable agriculture, buildings, and population to natural disasters [5, 23, 24].

South Carolina's educational achievement rates are lower than the U.S., ranking 36th of the 50 states (i.e., only 14 states have lower educational achievement rates) regarding people 25 years and older with high school degrees, 35th for those with college degrees, and 31st with post 4-year college graduate degrees. Six of the eight counties surrounding the Savannah River Site report lower educational achievement levels than the state, with only Lexington and Aiken counties having a higher proportion of high school graduates than the state.

As an illustration, we use two indicators to measure public educational base at the county scale: (1) proportion of population 25 and older without a high school education and (2) Niche's [25] rating of each county school system. The first is derived from the U.S. Census and published in EPA's EJScreen database [1]. The actual proportion is standardized to the state, with 100 being the state median rate. A number more than 100 means a poorer performance than the state. The second metric is a rating by Niche, Inc. [25], which rates communities on a scale from D+ to A+. The table also includes county-scale data regarding population change and broadband access. **Table 4** shows that Hampton, Allendale, Orangeburg, Bamberg, and Barnwell have high proportions of people without a high school degree and low Niche public school quality ratings, as well as marked population decreases and relatively low broadband access.

County	% Less than high school graduation, (state rate = 100)	Average school ratings by Niche	County population change, 2010–2020, %	proportion without broadband access, 2020, %
Hampton	168	C	−14.3	27.5
Allendale	166	D+	−19.4	33.1
Orangeburg	152	C+	−7.6	25.1
Bamberg	144	C+	−12.9	26.5
Barnwell	132	C+	−8.1	26.6
Edgefield	122	B	0.6	22.5
Aiken	108	B+	7.7	16.8
Lexington	82	A	15.4	12.8

(Data organized by county proportion of residents with less than high school education).

Table 4.
Educational achievement and public school ratings grouped by South Carolina County.

Regarding public education, in 2017, the State of South Carolina took over control of Allendale's public schools because of poor academic performance as it had done earlier from 1999 to 2007 [26]. Behind the terse summary that follows is the reality of massive differences in resources between the urban and rural areas; poor and more affluent areas; and areas with many and few people of color. The state of South Carolina ranked all its school districts [27]. The Superintendent of Education for South Carolina stated: "A millage tax in some of our poorest counties only brings in $20,000, and in our richest counties, it brings in $2 million." She then noted that it is so difficult to build a new school. At the top of the 10 school districts in South Carolina in need of support were Allendale, two in Bamberg, two in Barnwell, and one in Hampton. The Superintendent added that it would cost $1–2 billion to address the infrastructure needs of South Carolina's schools. We add that the five counties with the largest gaps in broadband access have the lowest public education rankings in **Table 4**.

Table 5 examines relationships between low educational achievement and demographic, health outcome, and population burdens for the 150 census tracts in the Savannah River region. The census tracts with the lowest educational achievement and low educational system ratings report higher asthma and heart disease rates, and

Variable	Zero-order correlations, R-values with low educational achievement
Energy burden	0.898
Heart disease	0.684
Asthma rate	0.853
Low income population	0.769
Population of color	0.689
Unemployment rate	0.487

Table 5.
Correlates of educational achievement in the study area (data represent calculations from census tracts).

a higher proportion of low income and people of color. They have higher unemployment rates and are stretched to pay their energy bills.

The public school system of this state needs to make a major investment in the infrastructure of its public schools, which might not be acceptable to some community school systems and the state government even if resources were to be offered. However, these data show the need. Earlier, we pointed out that it is to DOE's advantage to provide educational opportunities that will lead to potential employees and increasing local services for its employees and the site.

A crucial step in this direction would be for DOE to help provide increased science, technology, engineering, and mathematics (STEM)-related training in the counties with existing two-year technical Colleges and four-year colleges in the Savannah River region. This would require a smaller investment and would be focused on helping those having an interest and desire for a higher level education and/or technical training. Unfortunately, geographic disparities in terms of the locations of these higher education opportunities create greater travel burdens on many of those that would benefit the most. Aiken, for example, has a two-year technical college and a branch campus of the University of South Carolina. The Denmark Technical College, a Historically Black College or University (HBCU), is in Bamberg County but must also serve Allendale and Barnwell counties. It is the smallest of the schools serving the Savannah River site community with only 489 students. The City of Orangeburg in Orangeburg County has both a two-year technical college and two four-year universities. Both are HBCUs, one being the oldest private and the other being the oldest public HBCU in the state.

We calculated the number of higher education seats that are available per 1000 residents in each host county. We assumed that the current enrollments represented the number of potential seats available. In several instances, a regional technical college was designated to serve more than the county it was in, so we assumed that the total seats were available to each county.

Please note that our use of these data should not be taken at face value, because many of the residents are not going to go to college because of preference, family cost, and other personal reasons. Second, the seats numbers could change. For example, educational programs are increasingly delivered *via* the Internet, which may overcome physical seat shortages, assuming the availability of broadband, which as noted above is an issue in these counties. The point of this exercise is to demonstrate that there is a technical educational base in these areas for job training that could be delivered at the area's 2- and 4-year colleges.

Table 6 shows that Allendale, Edgefield, and Hampton counties have higher available seat rates per 1000 people than Lexington and Aiken counties. **Table 5** also shows higher available seat rates tend to be in the counties with lower rates of high school graduation and higher unemployment rates. Assuming that the potential seats estimates are reasonable, they indicate that there is existing capacity for an expansion of job-training and higher education opportunities in Allendale, Hampton, Orangeburg and elsewhere in this area.

Reliable and affordable high-speed internet connectivity is essential for economic activity throughout the US. Access to high-speed internet is vital for a diverse set of industries, including education, agricultural production, manufacturing, mining, and forestry, and it acts as a catalyst for rural prosperity by enabling efficient, modern communications between rural American households, schools, and healthcare centers as well as markets and customers around the world [28]. We believe that increasing entry-level higher education and technical training at the two- and four-year

County	Potential seats per 1000 residents	Population, 2022	Less than high school education, average of census tracts in each county	Unemployment rate, average of census tracts in each county
Allendale	177	7980	19.1	12.1
Edgefield	162	27,644	16.7	7.4
Hampton	119	18,844	17.9	8.5
Orangeburg	81	83,661	14.5	10.2
Bamberg	77	13,448	20.4	5.0
Aiken	34	175,141	12.4	7.3
Lexington	32	311,950	10.7	5.3
Barnwell	24	20,101	17.2	5.0

(Data organized by estimated seats per 1000 county residents).

Table 6.
Estimated seats per 1000 county residents in DOE-site region Counties.

colleges in this area requires improved broadband and increased computer access. The Biden Administration has made improving access to broadband a key element of its infrastructure programs [29]. In addition, the COVID-19 pandemic demonstrated the urgency of Internet access, as people relied on remote connections for medical visits, school, and work. Unfortunately, 22.3 percent of Americans in rural areas and 27.7 percent of Americans in Tribal lands lack coverage from fixed terrestrial 25/3 Mbps broadband, as compared to only 1.5 percent of Americans in urban areas. Approximately 182,000 households in South Carolina have no Internet access [30].

The lack of broadband access has disproportionally impacted lower income individuals who could improve their job prospects by taking remote courses to earn their GED or higher education credentials, as well as identify employment opportunities outside their local community. This also implies additional computers and tablets may be needed to take advantage of increased broadband access. The challenge of providing and maintaining Internet access in portions of this region is increased by the shrinking population in the rural and poorer communities noted above in **Table 4**. The cost of installing the necessary cable over large rural areas exceeds the potential revenue that can be earned by private operators.

The federal and state government will need to provide subsidies in these places. South Carolina's Office of Regulatory Safety [31] reported on a grant program to increase broadband access in rural Allendale County. Allendale, Bamberg, Hampton, Barnwell, and Orangeburg all have broadband gaps and declining population. Realistically, they need help from external sources to upgrade access and maintain it.

4. Conclusions

The current databases are an amazing improvement over what existed a decade ago. Barring a major change in government desire for information, we are confident that the databases presented here will be substantially updated. We expect the U.S. Congress to pressure U.S. federal agencies to work cooperatively and share software, hardware, and data. We predict that the data delivery systems featured here will be considered obsolete in a decade. A great deal of effort will be focused on quick access and the display of data.

These illustrations highlighted the needs of rural, poor, and underserved areas. Areas southeast of the Savannah River site have limited broadband access and a poor public school educational base yet possess the potential for educational outreach to disadvantaged communities through their existing two- and four-year local colleges. Also, while not addressed in the illustrations, these same areas have much higher natural hazard-related agricultural and population risk rates, along with higher levels of social vulnerability. The databases allow users to quickly go beyond anecdotal information and bring a good deal of credible data to identify and prioritize policy options.

Acknowledgements

Funding for the case studies summarized in this paper was from the Consortium for Risk Evaluation with Stakeholder Participation (funded through the Department of Energy (DOE-FC01-06EW07053) and Vanderbilt University. The authors are solely responsible for the contents of the chapter.

Conflict of interest

The authors declare no conflict of interest.

Author details

Michael Greenberg[1*], Henry Mayer[2], David Kosson[3] and Timothy Fields[4]

1 Rutgers and Vanderbilt University, Highland Park, NJ, United States

2 Vanderbilt University, Cape Charles, VA, United States

3 Vanderbilt University, Nashville, TN, United States

4 MDB, Inc., Washington, D.C., United States

*Address all correspondence to: mrg@rutgers.edu

References

[1] EPA. EJScreen: Environmental Justice Screening and Mapping Tool. 2022. https://www.epa.gov/ejscreen [Accessed March 13, 2023]

[2] EPA. EJScreen Environmental Justice Mapping and Screening Tool EJScreen Technical Documentation. 2022. Available from: https://www.epa.gov/system/files/documents/2023-01/EJScreen%20Technical%20Documentation%20October%202022.pdf

[3] Centers for Disease Control and Prevention (CDC). PLACES: Local Data for Better Health. 2023. Available from: https://www.cdc.gov/places/index.html

[4] Council on Environmental Quality. Climate and Environmental Justice Screening Tool. 2022. Available from: https://screeningtool.geoplatform.gov/en/about [Accessed March 13, 2023]

[5] Greenberg M, Mayer H, Fields T, Kosson D, Comments on Beta Version of the Climate and Economic Justice Screening Tool (CEJST) submitted to CEQ, April 22, 2022. Posted in Federal Register CEQ-2022-0002-0034, tracking number 12b-9185-gcc, April 26, 2022

[6] University of Wisconsin, Population Health Institute. County Health Rankings and Roadmaps. 2023. Available from: www.countyhealthrankings.org

[7] Agency for Toxic Substances and Disease Registry (ATSDR). The Environmental Justice Index: A National Tool to Measure the Cumulative Impacts of Environmental Burden on Health. 2023. Available from: https://www.atsdr.cdc.gov/placeandhealth/eji/eji-index.html [Accessed: March 13, 2023]

[8] Holm M. The Marshall Plan: A New Deal for Europe. Routledge, NY; 2016

[9] Hein C, Diefendorf J, Ishido Y, editors. Rebuilding Urban Japan After 1945. NY: Palgrave Macmillan; 2003

[10] Biggers J. The United States of Appalachia. Emeryville, CA: Avalon; 2006

[11] The White House. Justice40. A whole-of-government-program. 2022. Available from: https://www.whitehouse.gov/environmentaljustice/justice40/. [Accessed March 23, 2023]

[12] U.S. Government Accountability Office (GA). Environmental Liabilities: DOE Needs to Better Plan for Post-Cleanup Challenges Facing Sites. 2020; pp. 20-373. Available from: https://www.gao.gov/products/gao-20-373

[13] Markusen A. Sticky places in slippery space: A typology of industrial districts. Economic Geography. 1996;**72**(3):293-313

[14] Brauer J. U.S. military-nuclear material production sites: Do they attract or repel real jobs? Medicine and Global Survival. 1995;**2**(1):35-44

[15] Brauer J. Do military expenditures create net employment? The case of U.S. military-nuclear production sites. In: Brauer J, Gissy W, editors. Economics of Conflict and Peace. Aldershot: Brookfield, VT; 1997. pp. 201-226

[16] Hooks G, Getz V. Federal Investments and economic stimulus at the end of the cold war: The influence of Federal Installations on employment growth, 1970-1990. Environment & Planning A. 1996;**30**(9):1695-1704

[17] Bluestone B, Harrison B. The Deindustrialization of America: Plant

Closings, Community Abandonment and the Dismantling of Basic Industry. NY: Basic Books; 1982

[18] Russell M. Toward a Productive Divorce: Separating DOE Cleanups from Transition Assistance. Knoxville, TN: The Joint Institute for Energy and the Environment; 1996

[19] Greenberg M, Miller KT, Frisch M, Lewis D. Facing an uncertain economic future: Environmental management spending and rural regions surrounding the U.S. DOE's nuclear weapons facilities. Defence and Peace Economics. 2003;**14**(1):85-97

[20] Greenberg M, Isserman A, Frisch M, Krueckeberg D, Lowrie K, Mayer H, et al. Questioning conventional wisdom: The regional economic impacts of major US nuclear weapons sites, 1970-1994. Socio-Economic Planning Sciences. 1999;**33**(3):183-204

[21] Energy Community Alliance. Federal Budget Tracker. 2022. Available from: https://energy.ca.org/budget-tracker [Accessed July 11, 2022]

[22] OEM, DOE. Cleanup Sites. 2021. Available from: https://www.energy.gov/em/mission/cleanup-sites [Accessed May 22, 2021]

[23] Greenberg, M., H. Mayer, and D. Kosson. Environmental and Social Justice for DOE EM Site-Regions: A Geographical Analysis. Project Report, date. Vanderbilt University, Department of Civil & Environmental Engineering, VU Station B#351831, 2021

[24] Greenberg, M., H. Mayer, D. Kosson, and T. Fields. (2022) Economic, environmental, public health and demographic attributes of the U.S. DOE's major-site regions: A comparative analysis

[25] Niche. 2022. Available from: https://www.niche.com/places-to-live

[26] Bowers P. State Takes Over Allendale Schools- Again – in State of Emergency. The Post and Courier. 2017. Available from: https://www.postand courier.com/news/state-takes-over-allendale-county-schools [Accessed: August 18, 2022]

[27] Green M. 2022. South Carolina Spending Hundreds of Millions of Dollars to Help Schools with Aging Infrastructure. 2022. https://www.wistv.com/2022/06/09/south-carolina-spending-hundreds-millions-dollars-help-schools-with-aging-infrastructure/. [Accessed: August 27, 2022]

[28] U.S.D.A. e-Connectivity for all rural Americans is a modern-day necessity. 2022. Available from: https://www.usda.gov/broadband. [Accessed: August 24, 2022]

[29] NTIA, U.S Department of Commerce. Biden-Harris Administration Launches $45 Billion "Internet for All" Initiative to Bring Affordable, Reliable High-Speed Internet to Everyone in America. 2022. Available from: https://www.ntia.doc.gov/press-release/2022/biden-harris-administration-launches-45-billion-internet-all-initiative-bring

[30] Office of Regulatory Safety, South Carolina. Pilot Project Helps Expand Broadband Access in Rural Allendale. 2021. https://ors.sc.gov/news/2021-02-/pilot-project-helps-expand-broadband-access-in-rural-allendale-county [Accessed: August 18, 2022]

[31] South Carolina Digital Drive, State Broadband Office. Available from: https://www.scdigitaldrive.org/ [Accessed: September 29, 2022]

Chapter 4

Indoor Air Quality in Hospital Settings

Zemachu Ashuro, Gose Husen Washo and Kuma Diriba

Abstract

Many disease-causing microorganisms may have been introduced into the hospital's interior air by clients, staff, students, visitors, inadequate ventilation, or the outside environment. Hospitalized patients are at a greater risk of nosocomial infection as a result of enclosed/restricted space, overcrowding, and inadequate infection prevention and control (IPC) practices, which create a favorable environment for microorganism growth. Therefore, an institutional-based cross-sectional study was conducted to determine the indoor air bacterial load in different wards of the Hospital using passive air sampling techniques, and IPC compliance was evaluated using the World Health Organization IPC Assessment Framework (IPCAF) tool. In this study, the mean bacterial load ranged from 450±54.0 CFU/m^3 to 1585.83±155.64 CFU/m^3 after 60 minutes of culture media exposure. Gram-positive bacteria were the most commonly detected bacteria in hospital indoor environments, accounting for 51 (71%) of all detected bacteria. Fungi were found in 65 (90.3%) of the samples. The overall IPC compliance score in this study was 178/800 (22.25%), which was considered inadequate. The highest IPC compliance score in this study was 48%. Therefore, implementing IPC standards and regularly monitoring the bacterial load in the indoor air are essential for preventing the spread of microorganisms to visitors, patients, students, and healthcare workers.

Keywords: bacterial concentrations, hospital settings, indoor air quality, sedimentation plates, infection prevention

1. Introduction

Air pollution is referred to as a physical, biological, or chemical agent that pollutes the indoor or ambient (outdoor) environment and alters the inherent properties of the atmosphere [1]. The term "indoor air quality" (IAQ) means the air quality inside and surrounding buildings and structures, particularly in relation to the comfort and health of building occupants [2]. IAQ in healthcare settings is critical for patient safety and occupational health because healthcare professionals, employees, and clients spend extended periods of time in facilities [3, 4].

Hospital-acquired infections (HAIs) can be caused by pathogenic bacteria that can be found in healthcare facilities [5]. The Centers for Disease Control and Prevention (CDC) estimate that each year, nearly 1.7 million hospitalized patients acquire hospital-acquired infections (HAIs) while receiving treatment for other medical conditions and that more than 98,000 patients (1 in 17) die as a result of these infections [6].

Bacteria were found to be responsible for 90% of all HAIs. Bacterial indoor air quality reflects the sanitary conditions of the health facility. Bacteria, mold, and viruses can grow on ventilation system pans as well as the moist ceiling and floor [7]. Most bacteria may exist on dry surfaces for months and are resistant to disinfectants, which has an effect on patient health [8–10].

A lack of fresh air caused by increased building insulation, poorly maintained or operated ventilation systems, and poorly regulated temperature and relative humidity levels supports bio-aerosol presence and multiplication. Poor indoor air quality in developing countries may be caused by problems with design and inadequate ventilation [11, 12]. The presence of dirty attached toilets, insufficient waste disposal techniques, and an insufficient ventilation system all have an impact on the IAQ in healthcare facilities [13].

The majority of hospitals in developing nations lack an efficient IPC program as a result of a lack of knowledge, staff, water, laboratory backup, and safe practices among medical personnel [14]. The most prevalent disease-causing bacterial agents have been linked to poor indoor air quality and a variety of airborne infections [13, 15, 16]. The number of occupants, their activity, and the ventilation all influence the microbial load in hospital indoor air. Residents could be a source of microorganisms because bacteria are shed from the skin and respiratory tract. Gram-negative bacilli are found in sinks, washbasins, drains, nebulizers, humidifiers, and cooling towers [17–19].

The airborne colony count and IAQ parameters have significant associations; however, the association is not conclusive. Microorganisms can be affected by IAQ parameters [20]. Several studies in Ethiopia found a high risk of infection in hospital wards due to high bacterial loads in the air. Bacterial air quality was found to be above acceptable levels [21] in almost all of the hospital wards studied in Hawassa, Gonder, Jimma, and Adama [13, 22–24]. According to different research conducted in Ethiopian hospitals, the majority of hospital wards have a high bacterial concentration. However, none of them provide sufficient information on the various environmental conditions that contribute to high bacteria concentrations in indoor air. In addition, the WHO IPC Assessment Framework (IPCAF) and Hand Hygiene Self-Assessment Framework (HHSAF) are facility-level tools that each facility is expected to complete. Furthermore, the WHO IPC Assessment Framework (IPCAF) and Hand Hygiene Self-Assessment Framework (HHSAF) are facility-level tools that each facility is expected to complete. WHO encourages Ministries of Health to take the lead in promoting and coordinating the survey process and data collection among health facilities in their country (ideally through their national IPC focal point/team) [25]. However, no published data on the level of IPC compliance using WHO IPCAF tools were available in Ethiopia. Therefore, the main objective of this study was to assess IPC compliance at Dilla University Hospital using the WHO IPCAF tool, as well as determine bacterial concentrations in different hospital sites.

2. Methods

An institutional-based cross-sectional study was conducted at Dilla University Hospital in Dilla town, Gedeo zone, Southern Ethiopia, from June to August 2022, to determine indoor air bacterial load. A laboratory technician prepared blood agar according to standard operating procedure (SOP) one day before the data collection day, dispensed it into Petri dishes, and stored it in the refrigerator at 2-8°C after labeling it with the name of the media, preparation date, and expire date. We cleaned the sample collection area to avoid contamination during sample collection, and we decontaminated the cold box and transported it carefully to avoid contamination during transportation. To prevent contamination during incubation, we cleaned and decontaminated the incubator. The media for culture was prepared in accordance with the manufacturer's instructions or procedures, and sterility was verified by incubating a sample of the batch for 48–72 hours at a temperature of 35–37°C to observe for growth. Any media batches that showed signs of growth within 72 hours were discarded.

2.1 Methods of laboratory diagnosis

2.1.1 Gram stain

Gram staining was used to distinguish between gram-positive and gram-negative bacteria by taking a sample from culture after overnight incubation and staining it with Crystal violet, Gram's iodine, acetone alcohol (20 volumes of acetone to 19 volumes of methanol to 1 volume of water), and Safranin as a counterstain.

2.1.2 Microbiological analysis method

Air samples were collected two times a day, at 9:00 a.m. and 2:30 p.m. from different hospital rooms using a passive air method using 9 cm diameter Petri dishes filled with blood agar enriched with 5% sheep blood (Becton, Dickinson and Company) and dishes were left open using the 1/1/1 technique (1 meter from the walls, 1 meter from the floor, and for 1 hour), then covered with their lids and transported to the microbiology laboratory using a cold box for analysis. Colony-forming units (CFUs) were counted using a bacteria colony counter after each plate was incubated for 24 to 48 hours at 37°C under aerobic conditions. The CFU/m^3 was calculated using Omeliansky's equation after CFU [26, 27].

$N = 5ax10^4 (bt)^{-1}$, Where N = microbial CFU/m^2 of indoor air; a = number of colonies per petri dish; b = dish surface (cm^2); t = exposure time (min) [28, 29]. We incubated the fungal culture on Sabouroad dextrose agar medium for three days at 25°C. Gentamicin, chloramphenicol, and cycloheximide were added to Sabouraud dextrose agar to inhibit both gram-positive and gram-negative bacteria overgrowth, and cycloheximide was added to inhibit saprophytic fungi growth. After autoclaving and cooling the media to 45 to 50°C, all antibiotics were added.

2.2 Data collecting procedures for IPC compliance

The IPC compliance assessment data was collected by IPC-trained health professionals and the IPC coordinator at Dilla University Hospital using the WHO IPCAF tool [30, 31]. The following are the main components of the tool:

Core component 1: Infection Prevention and Control (IPC) program.
Core component 2: Infection Prevention and Control (IPC) guidelines.
Core component 3: Infection Prevention and Control (IPC) education and training.
Core component 4: Healthcare-associated infection (HAI) surveillance.

Core component 5: Multimodal strategies for implementation of infection prevention and control (IPC) interventions.

Core component 6: Monitoring/audit of IPC practices and feedback.

Core component 7: Workload, staffing and bed occupancy.

Core component 8: Built environment, materials and equipment for IPC at the facility level.

2.3 Standard definition

According to the WHO expert group, bacterial concentrations in indoor air must be less than 1000 CFU/m^3 is acceptable [32].

2.3.1 European Commission for nonindustrial premises sanitary standard for bacterial load

According to the European Commission, the sanitary standard of bacterial load for nonindustrial premises is classified as follows:

Very low (<50 CFU/m^3), Low (50–100 CFU/m^3), Intermediate (100–500 CFU/m^3), High (500–2000 CFU/m^3), and Very high (more than 2000 CFU/m^3) [33].

2.4 Data analysis

The data collection process was supervised by the principal investigator and co-authors, who also double-checked the collected data. The data were analyzed according to WHO guidelines. The maximum possible score was 800 because each core component of the IPCAF tool had a score of 100. IPC compliance was divided into four categories: inadequate (0–25%), basic (25.1–50%), intermediate (50.1–75%), and advanced (75.1–100%).

3. Results

In this study, we collected 72 indoor air samples from different hospital sites, and the pediatric ward had the highest indoor air bacterial count (1825 CFU/m^3), while the Neonatal Intensive Care Unit (NICU) had the lowest (390 CFU/m^3) after 60 minutes of culture media exposure time (**Figure 1**).

The mean bacterial load in the Neonatal Intensive Care Unit (450 ± 54.0 CFU/m^3), Orthopedics Ward (925 ± 136.37 CFU/m^3), and Emergency (903.75 ± 148.12 CFU/m^3) wards was within the WHO guidelines. However, the temperatures and relative humidity in all wards exceeded WHO guidelines (**Table 1**).

3.1 Indoor air bacterial load of hospital wards

According to the European Commission's nonindustrial premises sanitary standard, 58 (80.6%) of the samples in this study had high indoor air bacterial loads, and 8 (11.1%) had very high indoor air bacterial loads (**Figure 2**).

Gram-positive and gram-negative bacteria were found in this study, with gram-positive bacteria stained blue to purple (**Figure 3**) and gram-negative bacteria stained pink to red (**Figure 4**). According to the gram reaction, 71% was gram-positive and 29% was gram-negative. In 65 (90.3%) of the samples, fungal growth was observed.

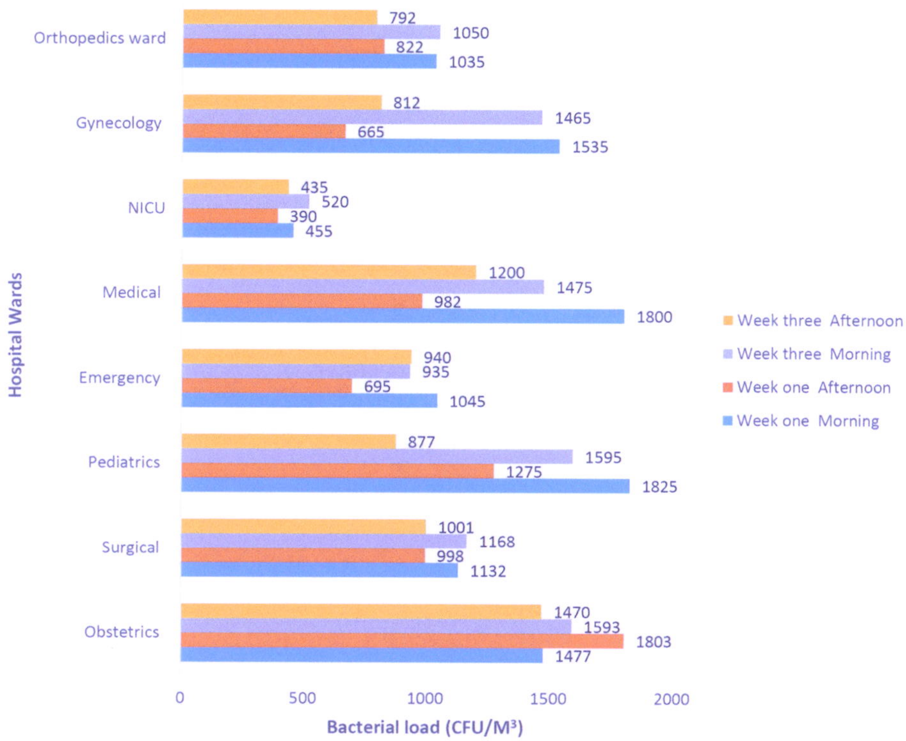

Figure 1.
Bacterial counts in air samples from different wards.

Wards/units	Bacteria (Mean CFU/m^3 ± SD)	Temperature (°C)	RH (%)	WHO guidelines
Obstetrics	1585.83 ± 155.64	27	61.1	Bacteria (<1000 CFU/m^3) Temperature (22–26.1°C) RH (30–60%)
Surgical	1075 ± 87.89	27.3	62.3	
Pediatrics	1393.12 ± 411.13	27.2	66.5	
Emergency	903.75 ± 148.12	26.5	61.2	
Medical	1364.37 ± 353.48	27.9	67.8	
NICU	450 ± 54.0	26.6	64.2	
Gynecology	1119.37 ± 444.53	28.2	62.9	
Orthopedics ward	925 ± 136.37	28.3	67	

Abbreviations: NICU: Neonatal intensive care unit; CFU/M3: colony-forming units per cubic meter; RH: Relative Humidity; WHO: World Health Organization; SD: standard deviation.

Table 1.
The mean bacterial concentrations, temperature, and humidity of different wards.

3.2 Infection prevention and control compliance

In this study, the overall IPC compliance score for six Dilla University Hospital wards was 178/800 (22.25%), which was considered inadequate. According to the

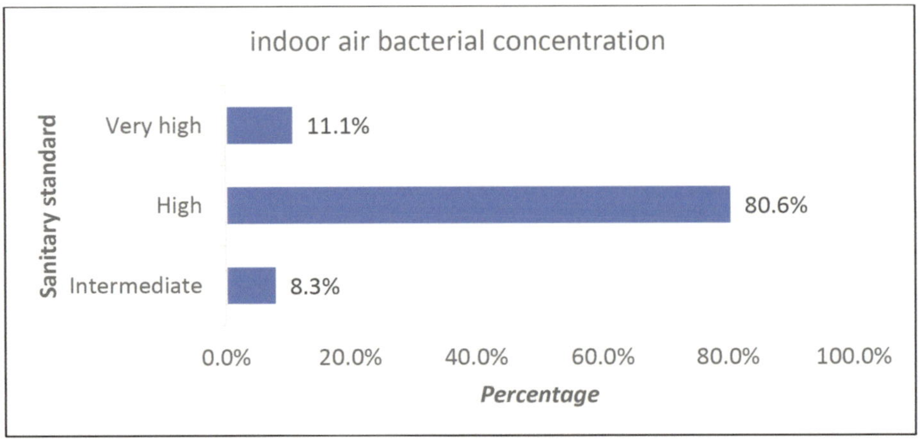

Figure 2.
Bacterial loads of indoor air.

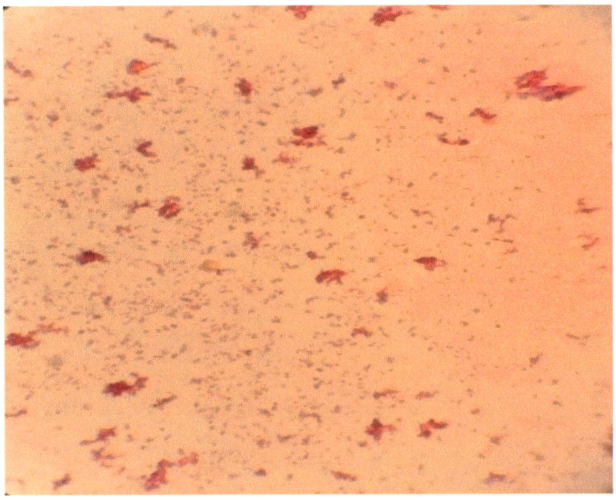

Figure 3.
Gram-positive cocci bacteria.

study's findings, the highest IPC compliance score was 48%, and the lowest compliance score was 0%. The majority of IPCAF tool scores ranged from 0 to 25%, indicating inadequate compliance. The core component "Built Environment, Materials, and Equipment" has the highest level of compliance, while healthcare-associated infection surveillance and multimodal strategies for IPC intervention have the lowest (**Table 2**).

3.3 Identified gaps in IPC activity implementation

The IPC compliance assessment result in **Table 3** revealed that there were gaps in implementing the IPC program and guidelines. There was no IPC team, the hospital's IPC program was not routinely supported by the microbiological laboratory, there were no guidelines for outbreak management and preparedness, and frontline healthcare workers were not involved in planning and execution of IPC guidelines. The strengths and identify gaps in education, training, and surveillance. IPC training

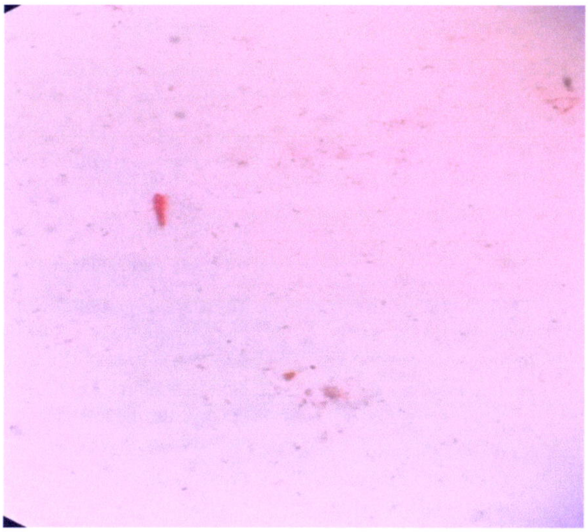

Figure 4.
Gram-negative rod bacteria.

IPCAF Core Components	Score	Percentage	Level of compliance
IPC program	35.0	35.0	Basic
IPC guidelines	25.0	25.0	Inadequate
IPC education and training	20.0	20.0	Inadequate
Healthcare-associated infection surveillance	0.0	0.0	Inadequate
Multimodal strategies for implementation of IPC interventions	0.0	0.0	Inadequate
Monitoring/audit of IPC practices and feedback and control activities	20.0	20.0	Inadequate
Workload, staffing and bed occupancy at the facility level	30.0	30.0	Basic
Built environment, materials and equipment for IPC at the facility level	48.0	48.0	Basic
Total score (Maximum 800)	178	22.25	Inadequate

Abbreviations: IPC: Infection Prevention and Control; IPCAF: Infection Prevention and Control Assessment Framework.

Table 2.
IPC compliance level of Dilla University hospital, southern Ethiopia, 2022.

was not frequently provided to healthcare workers, cleaners, patients, family members, and personnel directly involved in patient care. No surveillance was conducted for HAIs.

Multimodal strategies were not used to implement IPC interventions at Dilla University Hospital. There was no clearly defined IPC monitoring plan in place at the hospital. The WHO Hand Hygiene Self-Assessment Framework Survey was not conducted on a regular basis. The WHO healthcare worker-to-patient ratio was not

IPCAF Core Components	Strength	Identified gaps
IPC program	• The IPC focal person has dedicated time to IPC activities.	• There was no IPC team • The hospital's senior management does not show a strong commitment to supporting the IPC program. • The hospital's IPC program is not routinely supported by the microbiological laboratory. • A facility management professional was not assigned.
IPC guidelines	• The hospital has the expertise (in IPC and/or infectious diseases) to adapt guidelines. • Available hospital guidelines that are consistent with national/international guidelines.	• There are no guidelines for outbreak management and preparedness, prevention of surgical site infection, prevention of vascular catheter-associated bloodstream infections, hospital-acquired pneumonia, multidrug-resistant pathogens, and antibiotic stewardship. • Frontline healthcare workers were not involved in the planning and execution of IPC guidelines. • Healthcare workers did not receive specific training on IPC guidelines. • The hospital's implementation of the IPC guidelines was not regularly monitored.
IPC education and training	• IPC staff receive ongoing development/education (for example, by attending courses on a regular basis).	• The hospital lacked additional non-IPC personnel with the necessary skills to serve as trainers and mentors. • IPC training was not frequently provided to healthcare workers, cleaners, and personnel directly involved in patient care. • The administrative and managerial staff at the hospital did not receive general IPC training. • Periodic evaluations of the effectiveness of training programs were not performed. • There is no specific IPC training for patients or family members to reduce the risk of healthcare-associated infections.
HAIs surveillance	None	• No surveillance for HAIs
Multimodal strategies for implementing IPC interventions	None	• Multimodal strategies were not used to implement IPC interventions at Dilla University Hospital.
Monitoring/audit of IPC practices and feedback and control activities	• The hospital has trained personnel in charge of monitoring/auditing IPC practices and providing feedback.	• There was no clearly defined IPC monitoring plan in the hospital with specific goals, targets, and activities. • In the hospital, IPC processes and indicators were not monitored. • The WHO Hand Hygiene Self-Assessment Framework Survey was not conducted on a regular basis in the hospital. • There was no evaluation of cultural factors affecting hospital safety. • The reporting of monitoring data was not done on a regular basis.

IPCAF Core Components	Strength	Identified gaps
Workload, staffing, and bed occupancy at the facility level	• Bed occupancy at Dilla University Hospital was restricted to one patient per bed.	• In the hospital, the WHO healthcare worker-to-patient ratio was not maintained. • Wards in hospitals were not designed in compliance with international standards for bed capacity. • There is no adequate space of more than 1 m between patient beds in the facility. • No system in place in the hospital to assess bed capacity adequacy.
Built environment, materials, and equipment for IPC at the facility level	PPE was available in the hospital, in sufficient quantity, and for all uses for all healthcare employees	• There is no safe drinking water station for employees, patients, or families in any of the wards. • The majority of wards lack working hand hygiene stations. • No functional and adequate toilet facilities in the hospital. • There is inadequate artificial and natural functional ventilation in patient care areas. • No protected waste disposal pit and functional incinerator.

Abbreviations: HAIs: Healthcare-Associated Infections; IPC: Infection Prevention and Control; IPCAF: Infection Prevention and Control Assessment Framework.

Table 3.
Gaps identified in implementing the IPC program, guidelines, teaching, and training at Dilla University hospital in southern Ethiopia in 2021.

maintained in the hospital; there was insufficient space between patient beds, the majority of wards lacked working hand hygiene stations, there were no functional and adequate toilet facilities, no protected waste disposal pit, and no functional incinerator.

4. Discussion

The bacterial indoor air quality reflects the sanitary conditions of the healthcare facility. In this study, the indoor air bacterial concentration of Dilla University Hospital wards was found to be in the range of 390 CFU/m^3 and 1825 CFU/m^3. The findings of this study were higher than those of studies conducted at the University of Gondar Teaching Hospital in Northwest Ethiopia (480 to 1468 CFU/m^3) [13] and in Portuguese Hospital (240 to 736 CFU/m^3) [34] but lower than those of studies conducted at Jimma University Specialized Hospital (2123 to 9733 CFU/m^3) [22] and in hospitals in Dutse, Jigawa State (2770 CFU/m^3) [35]. This disparity could be attributed to differences in infection prevention and control (IPC) practices, temperature and humidity variations, traffic flow control mechanisms, and hospital settings. According to various literature, the main contributing factors for a high microbial load in the indoor environments of healthcare settings were temperature, relative humidity, and the number of patients and visitors [36, 37].

The highest mean indoor air bacterial concentration was found in the obstetrics ward, while the lowest was found in the Neonatal Intensive Care Unit (NICU) ward.

This study's findings were supported by a case study at Jimma University Specialized Hospital [22]. The high bacterial concentration in the obstetrics ward could be attributed to poor room cleanliness, overcrowding, and insufficient ventilation, the attachment of unsanitary latrines and shower facilities, and ineffective healthcare waste management.

The average indoor air bacterial load ranged from 450 ± 54.0 CFU/m^3 to 1585.83 ± 155.64 CFU/m^3. This study's findings were lower than the results of Jimma University Specialized Hospital, which ranged from 2123 CFU/m^3 to 9733 CFU/m^3 [22], but higher than those of a tertiary care hospital in India, which ranged from 65.52 CFU/m^3 to 1179 CFU/m^3 [11] and the University of Gondar Teaching Hospital in Northwest Ethiopia, which ranged from 480 CFU/m^3 to 1468 CFU/m^3 [13]. The high concentration of bacteria in the indoor air in this study could be attributed to poor healthcare waste management practices, overcrowding of wards, a lack of adequate artificial and natural ventilation, and poor sanitation of attached latrine facilities. According to the findings of various studies, poor ventilation systems can be a source of infections and can lead to the spread of various disease-causative agents or infectious pathogens [38].

In this study, a high percentage of the indoor air samples, 51.4%, exceeded the WHO expert group's standards. The findings of this study agree with those of the University of Gondar Teaching Hospital in Northwest Ethiopia [13] and the Hawassa University Comprehensive Specialized Hospital [24].

In this study, the majority of 58 (80.6%) of collected indoor air samples had bacterial concentrations higher than the European Commission's nonindustrial premises standard. Overcrowding, poor ventilation, unclean latrines, and splashes of blood or bodily fluids could all contribute to a high bacterial concentration. This study finding is supported by research from Nigeria [39], the University of Gondar Teaching Hospital in Northwest Ethiopia [13], and the Hawassa University Comprehensive Specialized Hospital Wards [24].

We detected both gram-positive and gram-negative bacteria after gram staining, but gram-positive bacteria were the most common, accounting for 51 (71%) of all bacteria detected. Similarly, studies conducted in hospital wards in Iran [40] and teaching hospitals in Nigeria [41] found that the majority of bacteria detected were gram-positive. This study's finding is higher than that of a study conducted in Hawassa, Ethiopia (43.1%) [42], but lower than that of studies done at Ayder Referral Hospital in Northern Ethiopia (87.3%) [43] and Felege Hiwot Referral Hospital in Northwest Ethiopia (81.6%) [16]. Possible causes for the high concentration of gram-positive bacteria in hospitals include dry conditions, spread through the nasal cavity and skin of healthcare providers, clients, and students at clinical attachments.

In this study, gram-negative cocci and gram-positive rods were the most commonly detected bacteria species. Similarly, studies in Dutse, Jigawa State [35] in Islamabad, Pakistan [44], and Portuguese Hospital found that both gram-negative cocci and gram-positive rod bacteria were commonly detected bacteria species in the hospitals' indoor environments [34].

Fungal growth was found in 65 (90.3%) of the samples in this study. This finding is supported by studies conducted in Nigeria [39], Northwest Ethiopia at the University of Gondar Teaching Hospital [13], and Hawassa University Comprehensive Specialized Hospital Wards [24]. The possible cause of high fungal loads in indoor air is insufficient artificial and natural ventilation, humidity, and temperature. Researchers demonstrated that effective hospital ventilation or filtration systems reduce indoor air fungal loads [38, 40]. Furthermore, the literature indicates that environmental factors such as humidity and air temperature contribute to a high fungi load in the hospital's indoor environment [40, 45, 46].

Proper practices of IPC measures can play an essential role in reducing hospital-acquired (nosocomial) infections. The findings revealed that the majority of core components of IPC were not practiced, and materials, guidelines, and equipment for IPC were not available at Dilla University Hospital. Six of the eight core components of IPC compliance had inadequate compliance, while the other two had basic compliance. The overall IPC compliance score for Dilla University Hospital in this study was 178/800 (22.25%), which was considered inadequate. This study's findings were lower than those of a study conducted at Lira University Hospital in Uganda, which found 28.5% [47].

PPE, detergents, and safe drinking water were among the IPC supplies that were limited in this study. The findings of this study are consistent with those of a study conducted in Ghana [48], a study conducted in the Arua district of Uganda [49], and the study conducted at Lira University Hospital, Uganda [47]. There is no IPC team at Dilla University Hospital, no budget has been allocated for the IPC program, the IPC program is not routinely supported by the microbiological laboratory, and no facility management specialist has been assigned. The findings of this study were supported by a study conducted at Lira University Hospital in Uganda [47].

5. Conclusion

Indoor air bacterial concentrations in the majority of Dilla University Hospital wards exceeded WHO guidelines and European Commission nonindustrial premises sanitary standards. Gram-positive rod bacteria and gram-negative cocci were found in this study, as well as fungal growth in 90.3% of the samples. Therefore, regular monitoring and evaluation of indoor air bacterial concentrations, as well as infection prevention and control measures, are necessary to control the introduction of microorganisms into the hospital. The overall compliance to IPC in Dilla University Hospital was 22.25% which was inadequate. The core component "Built Environment, Materials, and Equipment" and monitoring/surveillance have the highest level of compliance, while healthcare-associated infection surveillance and multimodal strategies for IPC intervention have the lowest. Therefore, the identified gaps in IPC implementation should be addressed in order to provide high-quality healthcare and reduce HCAIs. Furthermore, each room should be inspected on a regular basis to determine if there is any condition or situation that may enable microbial growth.

Author contributions

The study was conceptualized and designed by ZA. The data was collected, analyzed, and interpreted by ZA, KD, and GHW, and the book chapter was written by them. All authors reviewed and approved the final book chapter.

Funding

The Dilla University Research and Dissemination Office provided financial assistance for the completion of this study.

Conflict of interest

There were no potential conflicts of interest disclosed by the author in connection with the research, authorship, and/or publication of this article.

Ethical consideration

Before beginning the research, both verbal and written consent were taken into account. Letters of support from Dilla University and various stakeholders were also obtained.

Availability of data

Data will be provided upon request.

Author details

Zemachu Ashuro[1*], Gose Husen Washo[2] and Kuma Diriba[3]

1 Department of Environmental Health, College of Medicine and Health Science, Dilla University, Ethiopia

2 School of Medicine, College of Health Science and Medicine, Dilla University, Ethiopia

3 Department of Medical Laboratory Sciences, College of Health Science and Medicine, Dilla University, Ethiopia

*Address all correspondence to: zemash65@gmail.com

References

[1] Artiola JF, Reynolds KA, Brusseau ML. Chapter 18 - urban and household pollution. In: Brusseau ML, Pepper IL, Gerba CP, editors. Environmental and Pollution Science. Third ed. London, United Kingdom: Academic Press; 2019. pp. 311-326

[2] Kubba S. Chapter seven - indoor environmental quality. In: Kubba S, editor. Handbook of Green Building Design and Construction. Second ed. Boston: Butterworth-Heinemann; 2017. pp. 353-412

[3] World Health Organization. Regional Office for E. WHO guidelines for indoor air quality: selected pollutants. Copenhagen: World Health Organization. Regional Office for Europe; 2010

[4] Weikl F, Tischer C, Probst AJ, et al. Fungal and bacterial communities in indoor dust follow different environmental determinants. PLoS One. 2016;**11**(4):e0154131-e0154131

[5] Alemayehu T, Tadesse E, Ayalew S, et al. High burden of nosocomial infections caused by multi-drug resistant pathogens in pediatric patients at Hawassa university comprehensive specialized hospital. Ethiopian Medical Journal. 2019;**58**:45-55

[6] Klevens MR, Edwards JR, Richards CL, et al. Estimating health care-associated infections and deaths in U.S. hospitals. Public Health Reports. 2002;**122**:160-166

[7] Stockwell E, Ballard E, O'Rourke P, Knibbs L, Morawska L, Bell S. Indoor hospital air and the impact of ventilation on bioaerosols: A systematic review. Journal of Hospital Infection. 2019;**103**:175-184

[8] Jain A, Singh K. Recent advances in the management of nosocomial infections. JK Science. 2007;**9**:3-8

[9] Kramer A, Schwebke I, Kampf G. How long do nosocomial pathogens persist on inanimate surfaces? A Systematic Review. BMC infectious diseases. 2006;**6**:130

[10] Russell AD. Bacterial resistance to disinfectants: Present knowledge and future problems. Journal of Hospital Infection. 1999;**43**:S57-S68

[11] Srikanth P, Sudharsanam S, Steinberg R. Bio-aerosols in indoor environment: Composition, health effects and analysis. Indian journal of medical microbiology. 2008;**26**(4):302

[12] Onmek N, Kongcharoen J, Singtong A, Penjumrus A, Junnoo S. Environmental factors and ventilation affect concentrations of microorganisms in hospital wards of southern Thailand. Journal of Environmental and Public Health. 2020;**2020**:7292198

[13] Gizaw Z, Gebrehiwot M, Yenew C. High bacterial load of indoor air in hospital wards: The case of University of Gondar teaching hospital, Northwest Ethiopia. Multidisciplinary respiratory medicine. 2016;**11**:24

[14] Samuel SO, Kayode OO, Musa OI, et al. Nosocomial infections and the challenges of control in developing countries. African Journal of Clinical and Experimental Microbiology. 2010;**11**(2):102-110

[15] Ekhaise FO, Isitor EE, Idehen O, Emoghene AO. Airborne microflora in the atmosphere of an hospital

environment of University of Benin Teaching Hospital (UBTH), Benin City, Nigeria. World Journal of Agricultural Sciences. 2010;**6**(2):166-170

[16] Getachew H, Derbie A, Mekonnen D. Surfaces and air bacteriology of selected wards at a referral hospital, Northwest Ethiopia: A cross-sectional study. International journal of microbiology. 2018;**2018**:6413179

[17] Ayliffe GAJ. Control of Hospital Infection : A Practical Handbook. London: Arnold; 2000

[18] Gola M, Settimo G, Capolongo S. Indoor air quality in inpatient environments: A systematic review on factors that influence chemical pollution in inpatient wards. Journal of Healthcare Engineering. 2019;**2019**:1-20

[19] Weber DJ, Anderson D, Rutala WA. The role of the surface environment in healthcare-associated infections. Current Opinion in Infectious Diseases. 2013;**26**(4):338-344

[20] Hiwar W, King M-F, Shuweihdi F, Fletcher LA, Dancer SJ, Noakes CJ. What is the relationship between indoor air quality parameters and airborne microorganisms in hospital environments? A systematic review and meta-analysis. Indoor Air. 2021;**31**(5):1308-1322

[21] Pasquarella C, Pitzurra O, Savino A. The index of microbial air contamination. The Journal of Hospital Infection. 2000;**46**(4):241-256

[22] Fekadu S, Getachewu B. Microbiological assessment of indoor air of teaching hospital wards: A case of Jimma University specialized hospital. Ethiopian Journal of Health Sciences. 2015;**25**(2):117-122

[23] Shiferaw T, Gebre-silasse L, Mulisa G, et al. Bacterial indoor-air load and its implications for healthcare-acquired infections in a teaching hospital in Ethiopia. International Journal of Infection Control. 2016;**1996**:1-9

[24] Hailemariam M, Worku M, Azerefegne E. Intensive care units and operating rooms bacterial load and antibiotic susceptibility pattern. Journal of Surgery. 2016;**4**:60-64

[25] World Health O. Infection Prevention and Control Assessment Framework at the Facility Level. Geneva: World Health Organization; 2018. p. 2018

[26] Patricia G, Saravia S, Batistini P, Garcia Miniet M, Lavin P, Perdomo I. The quality of air at archives and the biodeterioration of photographs. International Biodeterioration & Biodegradation - Int Biodeterior Biodegrad. 2010;**64**:139-145

[27] Gutarowska B. Metabolic activity of moulds as a factor of building materials biodegradation. Polish Journal of Microbiology. 2010;**59**(2):119-124

[28] Fleischer M, Bober-Gheek B, Bortkiewicz O, Rusiecka-Ziólkowskaa J. Microbiological control of airborne contamination in hospitals. Indoor Build Environment. 2006;**15**(1):53-56

[29] Awad AH, Mawla HA. Sedimentation with the Omeliansky formula as an accepted technique for quantifying air borne fungi. Polish Journal of Environmental Studies. 2012;**21**(6):1539-1541

[30] World Health O. Guidelines on Core Components of Infection Prevention and Control Programmes at the National and Acute Health Care Facility Level. Geneva, Switzerland: World Health Organization; 2016

[31] Storr J, Twyman A, Zingg W, et al. Core components for effective infection prevention and control

programmes: New WHO evidence-based recommendations. Antimicrobial Resistance & Infection Control. 2017;**6**(1):6

[32] Nevalainen A, Morawaska L. Biological Agents in Indoor Environments. Assessment of Health Risks. Work Conducted by a WHO Expert Group between 2000-2003. Copenhagen, Denmark: World Health Organization; 2009

[33] Wanner H-U, Gravesen S. Biological particles in indoor environments: European Collaborative Action. Indoor Air Quality & Its Impact on Man. Report No. 12. Luxembourg: Commission of the European Communities, Directorate General for Science, Research and Development. Joint Research Institute - Environment Institute. 1993

[34] Cabo Verde S, Almeida SM, Matos J, et al. Microbiological assessment of indoor air quality at different hospital sites. Research in microbiology. 2015;**166**(7):557-563

[35] Mohammed B, Haruna I. Assessment of indoor air bacterial load and antibiotic susceptibility profile of bacteria from some hospitals in Dutse, Jigawa state. Bayero Journal of Pure and Applied Sciences. 2021;**12**:57-66

[36] Bhatia L, Vishwakarma R. Hospital indoor airborne microflora in private and government-owned hospitals in Sagar City, India. World Journal of Medical Sciences. 2010;**5**(3):65-70

[37] Qudiesat K, Abu-Elteen K, Elkarmi A, Hamad M, Abussaud M. Assessment of airborne pathogens in healthcare settings. African Journal of Microbiology Research. 2009;**3**(2):066-076

[38] Kumari DN, Haji TC, Keer V, Hawkey PM, Duncanson V, Flower E. Ventilation grilles as a potential source of methicillin-resistant Staphylococcus aureus causing an outbreak in an orthopaedic ward at a district general hospital. The Journal of Hospital Infection. 1998;**39**(2):127-133

[39] Wemedo S, Ede P, Chuku A. Interaction between building design and indoor airborne microbial load in Nigeria. Asian Journal of Biological Sciences. 2012;**5**:183-191

[40] Nasiri N, Gholipour S, Akbari H, et al. Contamination of obsterics and gynecology hospital air by bacterial and fungal aerosols associated with nosocomial infections. Journal of environmental health science & engineering. 2021;**19**(1):663-670

[41] Awosika SA, Olajubu FA, Amusa NA. Microbiological assessment of indoor air of a teaching hospital in Nigeria. Asian Pacific journal of tropical biomedicine. 2012;**2**(6):465-468

[42] Diriba L, Kassaye A, Yared M. Antibiotics susceptibility pattern of hospital indoor airborne bacteria in Hawassa university teaching and referral hospital, South Ethiopia. International Journal of Modern Chemistry and Applied Science. 2016;**3**(1):287-292

[43] Tesfaye T, Berhe Y, Gebreselassie K. Microbial Contamination of Operating Theatre at Ayder Referral Hospital. Northern Ethiopia; 2015

[44] Asif A, Zeeshan M, Hashmi I, Zahid U, Bhatti MF. Microbial quality assessment of indoor air in a large hospital building during winter and spring seasons. Building and Environment. Elsevier BV; 2018;**135**:68-73

[45] Park DU, Yeom JK, Lee WJ, Lee KM. Assessment of the levels of airborne bacteria, gram-negative bacteria, and

fungi in hospital lobbies. International Journal of Environmental Research and Public Health. 2013;**10**(2):541-555

[46] Chaivisit P, Fontana A, Galindo S, et al. Airborne bacteria and fungi distribution characteristics in natural ventilation system of a University Hospital in Thailand. Environment Asia. 2018;**11**(2)

[47] Opollo MS, Otim TC, Kizito W, et al. Infection prevention and control at lira university hospital, Uganda: More needs to Be done. Tropical Medicine and Infectious Disease. 2021;**6**(2):1-11

[48] Oppong TB, Amponsem-Boateng C, Kyere EKD, et al. Infection prevention and control preparedness level and associated determinants in 56 acute healthcare facilities in Ghana. Infection and Drug Resistance. 2020;**13**:4263-4271

[49] Wasswa P, Nalwadda CK, Buregyeya E, Gitta SN, Anguzu P, Nuwaha F. Implementation of infection control in health facilities in Arua district, Uganda: A cross-sectional study. BMC Infectious Diseases. 2015;**15**:268

Chapter 5

Community Engagement to Enhance Environmental Health Education to Reduce Communicable Diseases in Developing Countries

Benjamin Mwangi

Abstract

This chapter describes increasing and sustaining environmental health literacy (EHL) within the less disadvantaged and minority communities in third-world countries. People from developing countries experience systemic barriers to quality and affordable health due to economic disadvantages and lower educational attainment levels. Traditional cultural practices in developing economies reflect values and beliefs held by members for periods spanning generations. However, harmful conventional methods include female genital mutilation (FGM), forced feeding of women, early marriages, taboos, and religious beliefs that prevent women from controlling their fertility, nutritional taboos and traditional birth practices, early pregnancy, and bride price, among others. These undesirable practices affect public health negatively and increase the risk of otherwise preventable diseases. This chapter discusses community-based education approaches to promote healthy living styles and improve attitudes toward clinical interventions and treatments. The chapter contains examples of community-engaged education initiatives to promote EHL in various contexts, like community-initiated training that creates public awareness. Community-based education systems can contribute to building and sustaining equitable access to professional health and partnership between communities and stakeholders in the health sectors, emphasizing mutual co-learning and knowledge co-creation to meet unique existing and emerging needs.

Keywords: environmental health literacy, developing countries, sustainability, public education, and harmful cultural practices

1. Introduction

Communicable diseases refer to transferable diseases transmissible by contact with infected individuals, bodily discharge, fluids like respiratory droplets, blood or semen, and contaminated surfaces. The World Health Organization (WHO) defines communicable diseases as infectious conditions, including HIV/AIDS, tuberculosis (TB), malaria, viral hepatitis, sexually transmitted infections (STIs), and neglected tropical diseases (NTDs) [1]. Despite the success of vaccination programs worldwide, some infectious diseases like polio, malaria, TB, HIV/AIDS, and others constitute a significant health burden in most African countries [2].

Undesirable cultural practices, low levels of education, low income, and ignorance are among the key factors contributing to the spread of infectious diseases in African countries. WHO estimated that contagious diseases caused 14.7 million deaths in 2001, which accounted for approximately 26% of all global deaths [3]. However, WHO reports indicate that existing drugs and vaccines could have prevented these deaths [3]. Besides, food access and drinking water free from fecal contamination could have prevented approximately 2 million communicable disease-related deaths [3]. These challenges continue to undermine the quality of public health in developing countries despite the observed progress in controlling infectious diseases in developed nations. Low-income and lower-middle-income countries continue to experience the poorest overall health outcomes despite the progress achieved in fighting contagious diseases worldwide [4]. Although global interventions against infectious diseases have led to a two-fold reduction in HIV incidence between 2000 and 2018, the observed change is inadequate to reach the sustainable development goals (SDG) target to end the HIV/AIDs epidemic by 2030 [4]. Lack of focus on the cultural and social factors that increase the risk of infectious diseases in developing countries contributes to these slowed rates in reducing infectious diseases.

2. Burden and impact of communicable diseases in developing countries

Communicable diseases are infectious and preventable through appropriate lifestyles and sustainable health policies. Developed countries have made significant progress in eradicating infectious diseases from their populations. However, developing countries lag in eradicating infectious diseases. The situation increases the burden on public health. Failure to manage infectious diseases increases the burden of non-communicable diseases.

2.1 The burden of communicable diseases in developing countries

The burden of infectious diseases in developing countries remains a significant issue in health. Contagious diseases like respiratory infections, HIV/AIDS, diarrhea, Malaria, and tuberculosis claimed approximately 12 million lives annually [2] in developing countries in the past two decades. Infectious diseases contribute nearly 80% [2] of the disease burden in developing countries. The disease burden continues to increase despite the implementation of vaccination programs. Sub-Saharan Africa has the highest number of HIV/AIDS infections, which accounts for approximately two-thirds of the global population living with HIV [5]. Research findings from recent studies indicated that the cervical cancer burden caused by HPV infection was highest in Sub-Saharan African regions and Oceania, with more than 250 disability-adjusted life-years (DALYs) per 100,000 population in each area [6]. Due to undesirable cultural practices, the level of new infections in developing countries in Oceania and Sub-Saharan regions is higher than in developed countries.

Sub-Saharan countries continue to experience an epidemic of infectious diseases. Sub-Saharan Africa has approximately 37 million people living with HIV/AIDS, where groups with specific high-risk behaviors contribute to about 47% of new infections [7]. Some groups with high-risk behaviors, which contribute to the rise of new diseases, include LGBTQs, prisoners, drug addicts, and sex workers.

The ongoing interventions to reduce and combat the rise of infectious diseases fail to yield desirable outcomes. **Figure 1** shows HIV prevalence and antiretroviral therapy (ART) in some African countries. Countries like Eswatini, Lesotho, and Botswana have high levels of HIV infections and ART uptake. These outcomes suggest that the availability and use of ART interventions may contribute to the rising of new HIV infections. Despite ongoing interventions, cultural and social values are possible causes of the rising infectious diseases in developing countries.

2.2 Impacts of communicable diseases in developing countries

The lack of effective methods to manage infectious diseases in developing countries increases the overall public health burden. Okongo et al. developed a mathematical model indicating that TB and malaria treatment has an insignificant effect on HIV/AIDS prevalence [8]. The presence of HIV/AIDS increases the burden of diseases among high-risk populations. However, the mathematical models developed by Okongo et al. revealed that effective management of HIV/AIDS could lower the risk of developing other infectious diseases [8]. Ineffective ways to manage HIV/AIDS as an infectious disease in developing countries increase the burden of public

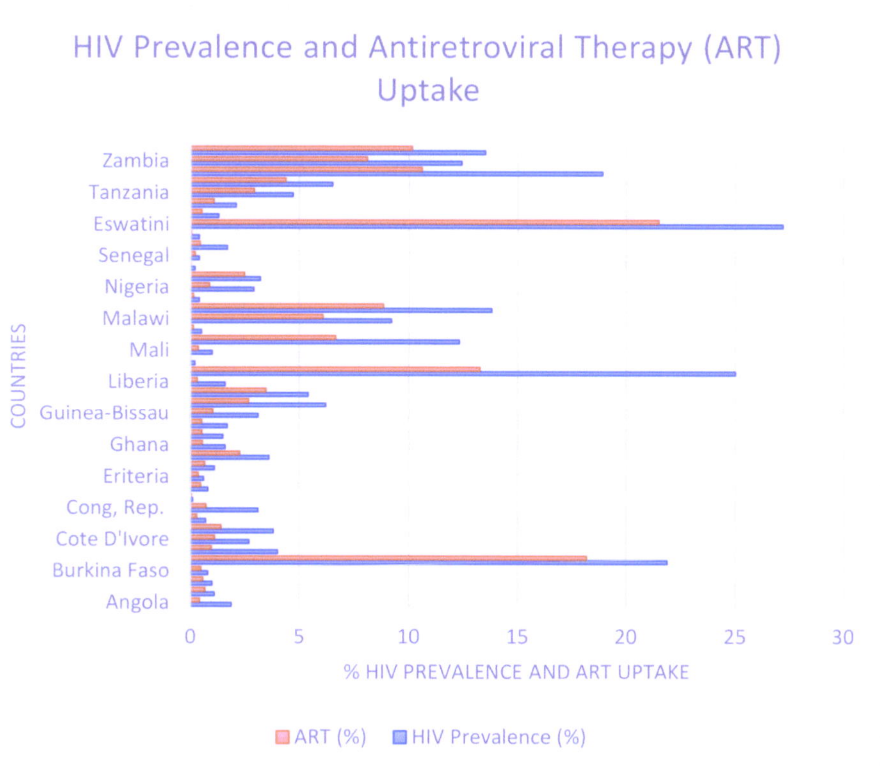

Figure 1.
HIV prevalence and ART uptake in different African countries. The data presented in this figure is a summary of the findings presented in Coetzee et al. ([5], p. 4).

health. The HIV/AIDS crisis at the end of the twentieth century and the resulting high burden of infectious diseases in low- and middle-income countries made managing infectious diseases a high-priority initiative [9]. Despite such intentions, ongoing interventions on infectious diseases are less effective because of low community engagement. Lack of public awareness in Sub-Saharan African countries leads to a situation where malaria and HIV/AIDS continue to drive substantial public health loss at higher rates than those recorded in the twentieth century [9]. Some risk factors for declining public health due to infectious diseases include inadequate knowledge and undesirable cultures that compel people to engage in unsafe lifestyles.

The ongoing epidemic of infectious diseases in developing countries increases the risk of non-communicable diseases. Sub-Saharan Africa faces a double burden of communicable and non-communicable diseases due to the adopted health systems and policies [10], which hinder the effectiveness of the adopted intervention. Sub-Saharan African countries lack robust health systems that can satisfy the needs of a population. Robust health systems integrate personal and public health care services, teaching and research, and health insurance [10]. The absence of practical research and health insurance policies in developing countries undermines the efforts to manage communicable and non-communicable diseases. The inevitable results include an increased burden in managing non-communicable conditions that people may fail to prioritize. Case study 1 presents a unique scenario of a woman struggling with non-communicable illnesses due to a lack of effective government measures to manage infectious diseases. Lack of adequate knowledge or access to appropriate preventive measures and ARVs contributes to Joan's deteriorating health. Joan's HPV and HIV/AIDS infections were the primary causes of cervical cancer. The increasing burden of infectious diseases exposes low-income earners in developing countries to higher risks of developing non-communicable conditions. HIV/AIDS infections increase the risk of developing specific malignancies [11, 12], which contributes to an emerging epidemic in Sub-Saharan Africa [13]. The less effective health interventions in developing countries are unsustainable because they increase the burden of sickness and the cost of treatment. For instance, failure to manage HIV/AIDS and HPV infections increases cancer risk in developing countries.

Case Study 1

Joan (anonymous name) is 48 years old and a single mother of two teenage girls. Joan is a sex worker in the City of Nakuru in Kenya, with an average monthly income of $300. Joan lives with HIV/AIDS and developed respiratory complications due to her working conditions. In addition, Joan developed cervical cancer due to a possible HPV infection. Neither she nor the two girls have received an HPV vaccine.

Joan did not have prior knowledge about HPV or effective prevention methods. Her income is inadequate to cater for reliable health insurance coverage. She cannot afford the required treatments for cancer and respiratory complications. The inaccessibility of Antiretroviral drugs (ARVs) exposes Joan to higher risks of deteriorating health. Joan struggles to raise her children and provide them with access to quality education. Her current health state leaves the two teenage girls to seek unreliable part-time jobs to sustain their needs.

Joan experiences familial rejection and social stigma as a sex worker. The African culture requires women to have and support a family. Unmarried women, especially sex workers, experience social and cultural stigma. The current social and cultural challenges discourage Joan from seeking assistance from non-governmental organizations.

The rising epidemic of HPV in Sub-Saharan African countries increases the burden of cancer cases. Various studies have reported a high prevalence of HPV infections in Sub-Saharan African countries [14–17], with high rates among men ranging between 19% and 100% [14]. These prevalence levels in Sub-Saharan African countries are higher than the global average, ranging between 1.3% and 72.9% [14]. The prevalence of HPV infections among African men contributes to higher infection rates among women. Results from a study, which comprised 1846 participants, indicated an average prevalence of 29.07% for women over 25 years, with the highest rate being 42.2% among women aged between 25 and 29 years [15]. Poor HPV management practices in developing countries contribute to the rising level of HPV infections and related cancer cases. Some barriers to effective HPV vaccination include limited health system capacities, socio-economic status, stigma, fear, and cost of vaccines [17]. These barriers lead to low levels of HPV vaccination among young girls and high cancer related cases at later ages. **Figure 2** shows data on cancer patients treated between January 2002 and May 2023 at Moi Teaching and Referral Hospital (MTRH),

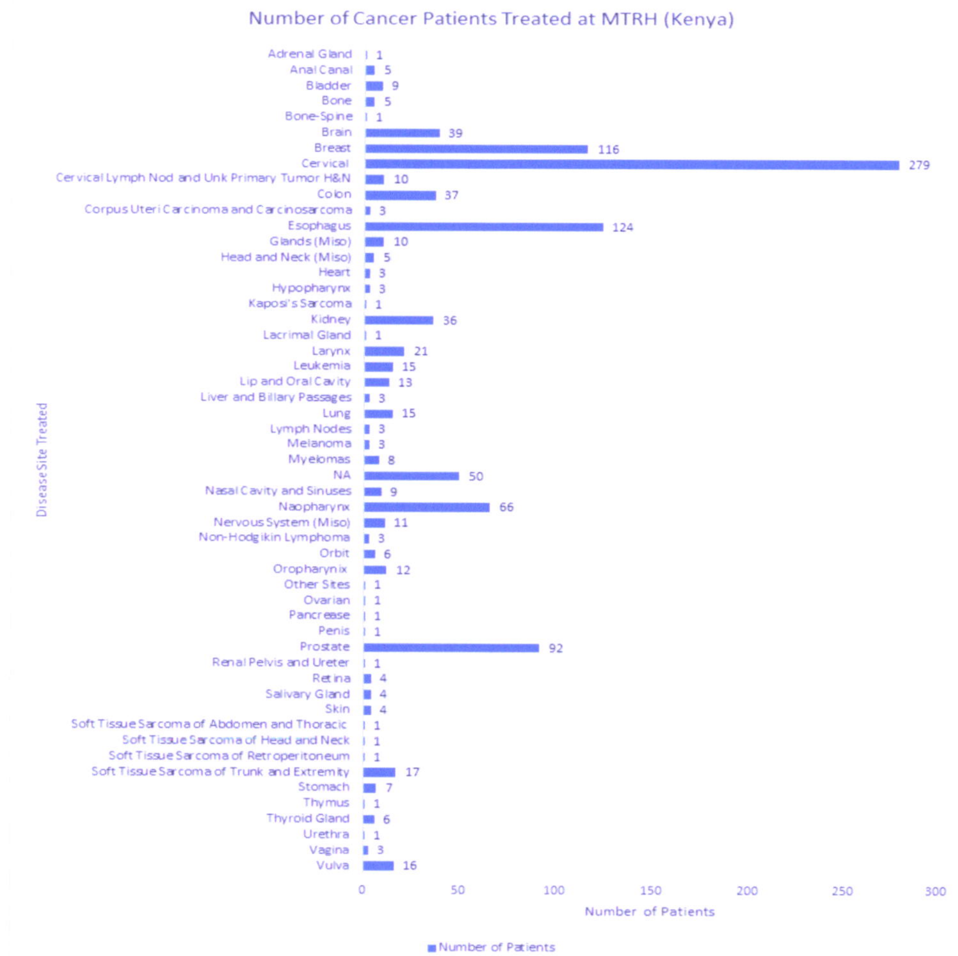

Figure 2.
Different cancer cases were treated at Moi Teaching and Referral Hospital between 1/1/2022 and 6/23/2023.

a radiotherapy center in Kenya. There were 279 cases of cervical cancer out of 1090 cancer patients treated at the facility within the stipulated period. Approximately 26% of all cancer cases treated at MTRH are cervical cancers, mainly caused by HPV infections. This data indicates the current scenario in Sub-Saharan countries where the lack of effective ways to manage infectious diseases increases the risk of non-communicable diseases. In addition, undesirable cultural and social practices are a significant factor that increases contagious diseases in developing countries.

3. Cultural factors that increase the risk of communicable diseases

Sab-Saharan African countries struggle with infectious diseases like malaria, HIV/AIDS, acute respiratory infections, cholera, tuberculosis, hepatitis B, Ebola, and COVID-19 [10]. Some of these infectious diseases occur due to specific cultural and social practices, which escalates the burden of public health. This section focuses on three contagious diseases and how cultural factors increase their risk in developing countries. Failure to align health interventions with socio-cultural values and practices through effective community engagement undermines their effectiveness.

3.1 Hepatitis

The prevalence of hepatitis infections occurs due to socio-cultural barriers to the utilization of appropriate sexual health services [18]. Cultural norms that influence people to underestimate preventative health, gender norms, and help-seeking behaviors increase the risk of hepatitis infections [18]. For instance, some cultural norms that promote male chauvinism may encourage men to engage in unhealthy sexual practices that increase their risk of hepatitis infections. Besides, the desire to fulfill specific cultural roles and values increases the prevalence of infectious diseases. Cultural and lifestyle practices that may include but are not limited to circumcision, female genital mutilation, tattooing, ear piercing, and unprotected sexual [19] activities increase the risk of hepatitis B virus (HBV) infections among teenagers. Some cultural practices dictate that people must engage in practices like traditional circumcision, which increases the risk of contracting HBV. Although Hepatitis B is a vaccine-preventable condition, its prevalence remains high in Ghana despite the introduction of vaccines [19]. Some religious and cultural practices discourage people from using pharmaceutical medications and vaccines, increasing the risk of infectious infections. Hepatitis B and C are significant public health problems in developing countries where between 40% and 80% of people ignorantly live with chronic hepatitis B and C [20]. Lack of knowledge of serostatus causes many infectious people to spread the virus to others. Inadequate public awareness of the importance of conducting regular health checkups and seeking timely treatment leads to a situation where contagious people spread the virus unknowingly.

3.2 HIV/AIDS

Social and cultural factors increase the prevalence level of HIV/AIDS in developing countries. Some undesirable cultural practices such as child marriage, socio-cultural gender, power, economic disparities, and sex at an earlier age [21–23] increase the prevalence of HIV/AIDS. The patriarchal culture in most African communities denies women equal opportunities for education, power, and employment and exposes them to early marriages. Several factors, including incentives to marry out young women to lessen the financial burden on low-income African families, contribute to child marriage [23]. Power disparities between men and women deny girls an opportunity to influence the decisions regarding their marriages. Besides, economic differences affect many girls to get married at an early age. These factors contribute to an increasing rate of HIV/AIDS infections. Some scholars [23] have found that the need to reinforce social ties, protect daughters from sexual adversity, and improve social status by marrying girls to well-off families is standard in African cultures. The lack of proper public awareness of how such practices impact health by increasing the risk of contracting HIV/AIDS is a significant problem in African countries.

Inadequate sexual and reproductive health and rights (SRHR) undermines the nature and responses to challenges that increase the risk of HIV/AIDS in African settings. Effective SRHR strategies require an extensive understanding of the socio-cultural and spatial settings where people live [24]. The relevant stakeholders can improve the quality of public health by engaging members of the target group to incorporate their cultural and social values. For instance, mitigating sexually transmitted infections (STIs) remains a significant challenge in Sub-Saharan Africa due to harmful cultural practices, illiteracy, and lack of access to screening services [25]. Most African women lack adequate knowledge of the impact of negative cultures on their overall health or the availability of appropriate health interventions. In addition, the fear of expressing pressing health concerns due to the imposed cultural values increases the risk of health burdens in African women.

3.3 COVID-19

COVID-19 represents a unique, infectious disease whose impact on Africans was influenced by socio-cultural values and norms. Mitigating the effects of the COVID-19 pandemic in a nonhomogeneous continent like Africa requires adopting locally relevant and culturally appropriate interventions [26]. Africans have unique and diverse cultures that influence their behaviors and attitudes toward health outcomes. The strategies used to contain COVID-19 in developed countries were less effective in Sub-Saharan communities depending on the targeted communities' cultural, social, and economic conditions. Failure to engage local communities leads to weak adoption of public health measures irrelevant to a cultural context [27]. These challenges became evident during the COVID-19 pandemic. For example, vaccine uptake hesitancy was a significant problem in Africa, which undermined the effectiveness of containing the pandemic [28–33]. Vaccine acceptance depended on people's interest in protecting against COVID-19, and concerns about possible side effects were the leading cause of hesitancy [31]. Lack of adequate education on the effectiveness of vaccines in containing a pandemic influences people to disregard the containment measures taken by governments and healthcare institutions. Positioning vaccines to reflect equitable access and benefits to the targeted population effectively reduces possible resistance [28]. Failure to engage community leaders and local healthcare providers in rolling out vaccination programs contributed to the hesitancy observed across developing countries. For instance, some Africans regarded compulsory isolation and vaccination as violating their fundamental rights to association, religion, and freedom of choice. The hesitancy to uptake COVID-19 indicated people's desire to safeguard their independence and participate fully in deciding the right health interventions that align with their needs.

The case study of Tanzania in managing COVID-19 reveals the impact of cultural practices in increasing the risk of infectious diseases. The negative perception toward foreign COVID-19 vaccines compelled Tanzanians to use plant products like eucalyptus species, pepper, berries, ginger, garlic, and onions, among others, to manage the pandemic [34]. Although the natural products may have had positive outcomes in containing the pandemic, the desire to safeguard cultural independence compelled Tanzanians to reject pharmaceutical vaccines. **Figure 3** shows some methods used to control the COVID-19 pandemic in Tanzania, despite the need for adequate scientific evidence regarding their effectiveness.

Women from North-West Tanzania gave accounts of how they used cultural-based containment measures to control the COVID-19 pandemic. Some of their interventions included biomedical solutions, cultural and religious frames, traditional practices, and spiritual interventions alongside public health recommendations [35]. Such patterns reveal the importance of cultural and religious values in promoting public health. Excluding important socio-cultural values in the adopted interventions may

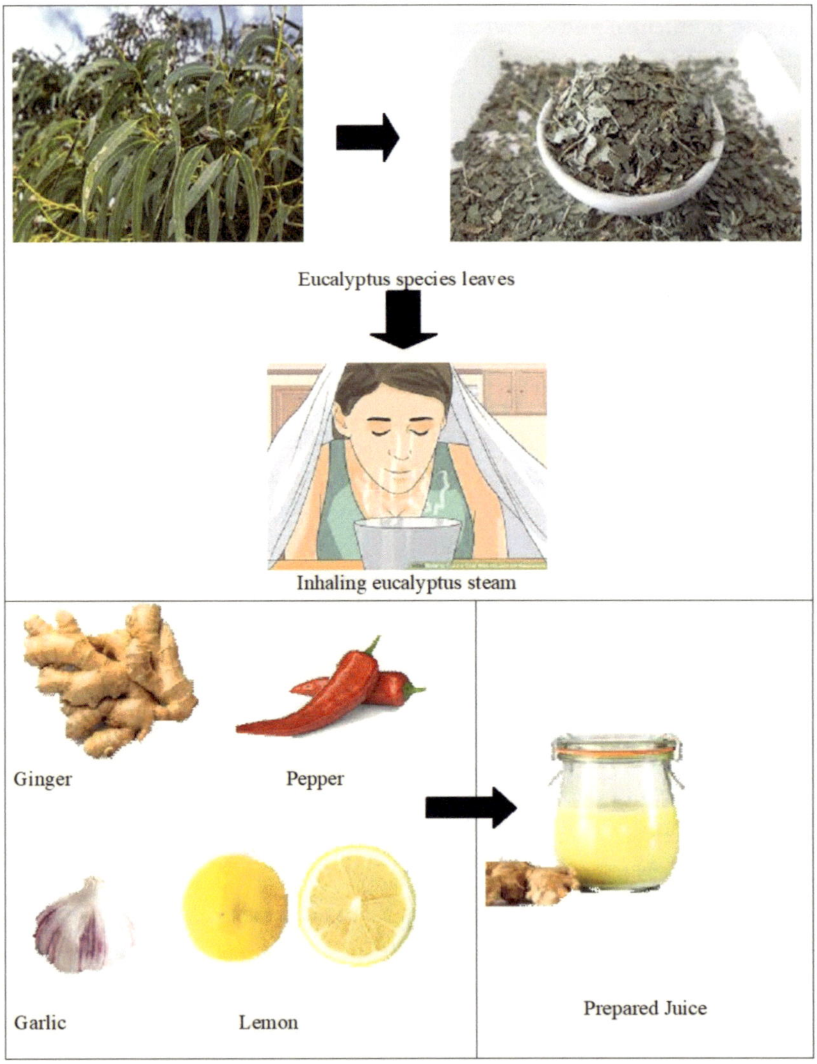

Figure 3.
Natural products used to control the COVID-19 pandemic in Tanzania. Modification of a chart presented in Mlozi ([34], p. 3).

result in hesitancy to adopt recommended public health interventions. The introduction of various concoctions to curb the COVID-19 pandemic in Tanzania resulted from the experience of using medicinal herbs to prevent, treat, and cure epidemics in the past [36]. Traditional medicine practices and interventions are crucial in enhancing and promoting public health. In addition, religious and spiritual practices accompanying such conventional health interventions are essential in promoting public acceptance of proposed medications. Although extensive use of scientifically unproved interventions may increase the prevalence level of infectious diseases, the case study of Tanzania provides a renewed perception of managing communicable diseases.

4. The role of community education in minimizing the risk of communicable diseases

Community education is essential in promoting health sustainability by minimizing the risk of infectious diseases. Educational instructions through face-to-face or online approaches were critical to promoting public health during the COVID-19 pandemic [37]. Engaging people through relevant education and instructions can allow them to understand the importance of embracing scientifically proven health interventions. Such practices promote sustainability by ensuring the effective use of available resources for prompting public health due to reduced hesitancy in adopting pharmaceutical medications. Education allows people to develop a wide range of skills and behaviors that can predispose them toward improved health and well-being [38]. Public health education must motivate people to change their lifestyles and behaviors to promote health outcomes. Effective community education programs should focus on addressing the existing gaps in a specific community. For instance, a general lack of knowledge and misconceptions about the transmission of infectious diseases is a current problem [39]. Healthcare workers should strive to understand people's misconceptions about a particularly contagious disease. The designed learning interventions should incorporate adequate knowledge to allow people to embrace preventive measures for infectious diseases and their valued socio-cultural practices and beliefs. Healthcare providers should understand the importance of socio-cultural values in a community to avoid people resisting the appropriate ways of controlling infectious diseases. Effective community education should involve collaboration between primary care providers (PCPs) and patients. Some elderly HIV/AIDS patients expressed their concerns that PCPs lack an understanding of their sexual needs [39]. Taking time to understand the factors that affect health perceptions among specific groups can reduce resistance and negligence among the target groups.

Community education programs should align with the local socio-cultural needs of the targeted communities. Most developing countries have cultural diversity, influencing people's behaviors and attitudes toward infectious diseases. For example, outreach programs in Vietnam effectively reduced risky sexual behaviors and increased HIV-testing services among the targeted high-risk groups [40]. Aligning communicable disease intervention programs with local community cultures can produce positive reception. People can appreciate the importance of various mitigations and embrace them as effective living methods to lower their risk of contracting infectious diseases. This intervention is applicable in communities where people engage in health-risk cultural practices like traditional circumcision, FGM, early marriages, and polygamous marriages. Engaging people in learning the health risks associated with valued cultural practices that promote infectious diseases can influence them to adopt healthy ways of living that lower the burden of infectious diseases.

Community education programs should incorporate cultural and social beliefs in the target population. The case of Tanzania reveals the need to allow people to combine their cultural values into the health interventions used to control infectious diseases. People attach more significant meaning to traditional, religious, and spiritual practices, influencing their overall health outcomes. Healthcare providers should engage community members in developing countries in developing community engagement health programs.

5. Conclusion

Communicable diseases continue to impose a significant health burden on public health systems in developing countries. Lack of effective community education increases the risk of communicable diseases in developing countries. Community education is essential in promoting health sustainability by reducing the risk of infectious diseases. Effective community education programs should align with the local socio-cultural needs of the targeted communities. Such interventions should integrate cultural diversity, influencing people's behaviors and attitudes toward infectious diseases.

Acknowledgements

I acknowledge my dear wife Vivian Wanjiru and children, Dan Ndashi, Ann Muthoni, Ruth Waithera, Joseph Mwangi, Naomi Wanjiru for their support throughout this project. I also acknowledge their moral support and their willingness to give me ample time.

Acronyms and abbreviations

EHL	environmental health literacy
FGM	female genital mutilation
WHO	World Health Organization
TB	tuberculosis
STIs	sexually transmitted infections
NTDs	neglected tropical diseases
SDG	sustainable development goals
DALYs	disability-adjusted life-years
ART	antiretroviral therapy
MTRH	Moi Teaching and Referral Hospital
HBV	hepatitis B virus
SRHR	sexual and reproductive health and rights
PCPs	primary care providers

Author details

Benjamin Mwangi
Nakuru Regional Cancer Centre, Nairobi, Kenya

*Address all correspondence to: benjaminmwangi@mtrh.go.ke

References

[1] World Health Organization. Our Work: Communicable and Non-communicable Diseases, and Mental Health. Geneva, Switzerland: WHO; 2023. Available from: https://www.who.int/our-work/communicable-and-noncommunicable-diseases-and-mental-health

[2] Boutayeb A, Boutayeb S. The burden of non-communicable diseases in developing countries. International Journal for Equity in Health. 2005;**4**(1):532-544. DOI: 10.1186/1475-9276-4-2

[3] Kindhauser MK. Global Defence against the Infectious Disease Threat. Geneva, Switzerland: World Health Organization; 2003

[4] World Health Organization. World Health Statistics 2020: Monitoring Health SDGs. Baltimore, Maryland; 2020

[5] Coetzee L, Bogler L, De Neve J, Bärnighausen T, Geldsetzer P, Vollmer S. HIV antiretroviral therapy and non-communicable diseases in sub-Saharan Africa: Empirical evidence from 44 countries over the period 2000 to 2016. Journal of the International AIDS Society. 2019;**22**(7):1-7. DOI: 10.1002/jia2.25364

[6] Coates MM et al. Burden of non-communicable diseases from infectious causes in 2017: A modelling study. The Lancet Global Health. 2020;**8**:e1489-e1498. DOI: 10.1016/S2214-109X(20)30358-2

[7] Achwoka D, Mutave R, Oyugi JO, Achia T. Tackling an emerging epidemic: The burden of non-communicable diseases among people living with HIV/AIDS in sub-Saharan Africa. Pan African Medical Journal. 2020;**36**(271):1-9. DOI: 10.11604/pamj.2020.36.271.22810

[8] Okongo MO, Lunani MA, Menge BK, Ochwach JO. The impact of HIV/AIDS treatment and counseling on the prevalence of tuberculosis and malaria Co-infections. International Journal of Mathematical Analysis. 2023;**17**(2):51-67. DOI: 10.12988/ijma.2023.511270

[9] Zeltner T, Riahi F, Huber J. Acute and chronic health challenges in sub-Saharan Africa: An unfinished agenda. In: Africa's Population: In Search of a Demographic Dividend. 2017. pp. 283-297. DOI: 10.1007/978-3-319-46889-1_18

[10] Sarpong E et al. Zero malaria: A mirage or reality for populations of sub-Saharan Africa in health transition. Malaria Journal. 2022;**21**(1):1-12. DOI: 10.1186/s12936-022-04340-1

[11] National Cancer Institute. HIV Infection and Cancer Risk. Bethesda, Maryland: National Cancer Institute; 2017. Available from: https://www.cancer.gov/about-cancer/causes-prevention/risk/infectious-agents/hiv-fact-sheet

[12] Oliver NT, Chiao EY. Malignancies in women with HIV infection. Current Opinion in HIV and AIDS. 2017;**12**(1):69-76. DOI: 10.1097/coh.0000000000000332

[13] Sasco AJ et al. The challenge of AIDS-related malignancies in sub-Saharan Africa. PLoS One. 2010;**5**(1):1-10. DOI: 10.1371/journal.pone.0008621

[14] Olesen TB, Munk C, Christensen J, Andersen KK, Kjaer SK. Human papillomavirus prevalence among men in sub-Saharan Africa: A systematic review and meta-analysis. Sexually Transmitted Infections. 2014;**90**(6):455-462. DOI: 10.1136/sextrans-2013-051456

[15] Mutombo AB, Benoy I, Tozin R, Bogers J, Van geertruyden J-P, Jacquemyn Y. Prevalence and distribution of human papillomavirus genotypes among women in Kinshasa, the Democratic Republic of the Congo. Journal of Global Oncology. 2019;**5**:1-9. DOI: 10.1200/jgo.19.00110

[16] Okoye JO, Ofodile CA, Adeleke OK, Obioma O. Prevalence of high-risk HPV genotypes in sub-Saharan Africa according to HIV status: A 20-year systematic review. Epidemiology and Health. 2021;**43**:1-11. DOI: 10.4178/epih.e2021039

[17] Kutz J-M, Rausche P, Gheit T, Puradiredja DI, Fusco D. Barriers and facilitators of HPV vaccination in sub-Saharan Africa: A systematic review. BMC Public Health. 2023;**23**(1):1-13. DOI: 10.1186/s12889-023-15842-1

[18] Ghimire S, Hallett J, Gray C, Lobo R, Crawford G. What works? Prevention and control of sexually transmitted infections and blood-borne viruses in migrants from sub-Saharan Africa, Northeast Asia and Southeast Asia living in high-income countries: A systematic review. International Journal of Environmental Research and Public Health. 2019;**16**(7): 1-17. DOI: 10.3390/ijerph16071287

[19] Nyambah PK, Adjei R, Sarfo B. Seroprevalence of hepatitis B virus infection is associated with male circumcision among senior high school students in the Krachi Nchumuru District in the Oti region of Ghana: A cross-sectional study. Research Square. 2023:1-22. DOI: 10.21203/rs.3.rs-2845421/v1 [Pre-print]

[20] Ayele A, Abera D, Hailu M, Birhanu M, Desta K. Prevalence and associated risk factors for hepatitis B and C viruses among refugees in Gambella, Ethiopia. BMC Public Health. 2020;**20**(1):1-10. DOI: 10.1186/s12889-020-08893-1

[21] Obeagu EI, Alum EU, Obeagu GU. Factors associated with prevalence of HIV among youths: A review of Africa perspective. Madonna University Journal of Medicine and Health Sciences. 2023;**3**(1):13-18

[22] Mhungu A, Sixsmith J, Burnett E. Adolescent girls and young Women's experiences of living with HIV in the context of patriarchal culture in sub-Saharan Africa: A scoping review. AIDS and Behavior. 2022;**27**:1365-1379. DOI: 10.1007/s10461-022-03872-6

[23] Yaya S, Odusina EK, Bishwajit G. Prevalence of child marriage and its impact on fertility outcomes in 34 sub-Saharan African countries. BMC International Health and Human Rights. 2019;**19**(1):1-11. DOI: 10.1186/s12914-019-0219-1

[24] Wado YD, Bangha M, Kabiru CW, Feyissa GT. Nature of, and responses to key sexual and reproductive health challenges for adolescents in urban slums in sub-Saharan Africa: A scoping review. Reproductive Health. 2020;**17**(1):1-14. DOI: 10.1186/s12978-020-00998-5

[25] Armstrong-Mensah EA, Ebiringa D-P, Whitfield K, Coldiron J. Genital chlamydia trachomatis infection: Prevalence, risk factors and adverse pregnancy and birth outcomes in children and women in sub-Saharan Africa. International Journal of Maternal and Child Health and AIDS (IJMA). 2021;**10**(2):251-257. DOI: 10.21106/ijma.523

[26] Renzaho AMN. The need for the right socio-economic and cultural fit in the COVID-19 response in sub-Saharan Africa: Examining demographic, economic political, health, and socio-cultural differentials in COVID-19 morbidity and mortality. International Journal of Environmental Research and Public Health. 2020;**17**(10):1-14. DOI: 10.3390/ijerph17103445

[27] Aduh U et al. Risk perception, public health interventions, and Covid-19 pandemic control in sub-Saharan Africa. Journal of Public Health in Africa. 2020;**21**(1562):1-16. DOI: 10.4081/jphia.2021.1622

[28] Mutombo PN et al. COVID-19 vaccine hesitancy in Africa: A call to action. The Lancet Global Health. 2021;**10**(3):e320-e321. DOI: 10.1016/s2214-109x(21)00563-5

[29] Sallam M. COVID-19 vaccine hesitancy worldwide: A concise systematic review of vaccine acceptance rates. Vaccine. 2021;**9**(2):1-14. DOI: 10.3390/vaccines9020160

[30] Aborode AT et al. Vaccine hesitancy in Africa: Causes and strategies to the rescue. Therapeutic Advances in Vaccines and Immunotherapy. 2021;**9**:1-5. DOI: 10.1177/25151355211047514

[31] Machingaidze S, Wiysonge CS. Understanding COVID-19 vaccine hesitancy. Nature Medicine. 2021;**27**(27):1338-1339. DOI: 10.1038/s41591-021-01459-7

[32] Afolabi AA, Ilesanmi OS. Dealing with vaccine hesitancy in Africa: The prospective COVID-19 vaccine context. Pan African Medical Journal. 2021;**38**:1-7. DOI: 10.11604/pamj.2021.38.3.27401

[33] Cooper S, van Rooyen H, Wiysonge CS. COVID-19 vaccine hesitancy in South Africa: How can we maximize uptake of COVID-19 vaccines? Expert Review of Vaccines. 2021;**20**(8):1-13. DOI: 10.1080/14760584.2021.1949291

[34] Mlozi SH. The role of natural products from medicinal plants against COVID-19: Traditional medicine practice in Tanzania. Heliyon. 2022;**8**(6):1-6. DOI: 10.1016/j.heliyon.2022.e09739

[35] Mchome Z, Mshana G, Peter E, Aloyce D, Kapiga S, Stöckl H. Women's narratives about COVID-19, preventive practices and sources of information in northwestern Tanzania. International Journal of Environmental Research and Public Health. 2021;**18**(10):1-13. DOI: 10.3390/ijerph18105261

[36] Kamazima SR, Kakoko DCV, Kazaura M. "Manifold tactics are used to control and prevent pandemics in contemporary Africa": A case of Tanzania's fight against COVID-19. International Journal of Advanced Scientific Research and Management. 2020;**5**(11):20-33. DOI: 10.36282/ijasrm/5.11.2020.1770

[37] Honein MA. Summary of guidance for public health strategies to address high levels of community transmission of SARS-CoV-2 and related deaths, December 2020. MMWR. Morbidity and Mortality Weekly Report. 2020;**69**:1860-1867. DOI: 10.15585/mmwr.mm6949e2

[38] Raghupathi V, Raghupathi W. The influence of education on health: An empirical assessment of OECD countries for the period 1995-2015. Archives of Public Health. 2020;**78**(1):1-18. DOI: 10.1186/s13690-020-00402-5

[39] Davis TEK, Elder MA. HIV knowledge and preferences for HIV prevention among older adults living in the community. Gerontology and Geriatric Medicine. 2020;**6**:1-10. DOI: 10.1177/2333721420927948

[40] Sabin LL et al. Effectiveness of community outreach HIV prevention programs in Vietnam: A mixed methods evaluation. BMC Public Health. 2019;**19**(1):1-17. DOI: 10.1186/s12889-019-7418-5

Chapter 6

Poor Disposal of Soiled Diapers in Sub-Saharan Africa: A Gap in Environmental Health Literacy in Rural Communities

Lutendo Sylvia Mudau, Ayanda Myranda Derby Thumbathi and Davies Veli Nkosi

Abstract

Disposable diapers are designed to absorb and retain a baby's urine and fecal matter whilst keeping their skin dry and healthy. Although they are convenient and a huge benefit in today's busy life-style, their impact on the environment is becoming unbearable due to poor handling and disposal practices. Disposable diapers are known to reduce the burden of domestic chores for many care-givers. However, the threat to environmental and public health due to its ability to contaminate water and land cannot be ignored. These practices show a serious gap in Environmental Health Literacy (EHL) within the communities of Sub-Saharan Africa (SSA). Seemingly, more than 95% of these communities use disposable diapers with limited knowledge on how to dispose of them and protect the environment. Apparently, there are no programs in place to transfer knowledge to care-givers on how to prevent an impact on the environment after use. On the other hand, there is no regulation or procedure in place focusing on practices and disposal. As a result, inappropriate handling and disposal continue to be a public health risk to communities, with less appropriate measures to prevent environmental and health risks.

Keywords: environmental health literacy, soiled disposable diapers, environmental impact, health impact, environmental health assessment, open defecation, public health

1. Introduction

Environmental Health Literacy (EHL) is a concept that integrates environmental and health literacy, with the aim of developing self-empowering skills and the competency required to make an informed choice to reduce health risks and enhance environmental protection [1]. The use and disposal of soiled diapers in rural areas represent a lack of Environmental Health Literacy. This is usually observed in disadvantaged communities with low socio-economic status, and lack of environmental health risks awareness programs [2]. In Sub-Saharan Africa (SSA), especially in the rural areas, waste management has become a serious challenge. This is evident in most areas where communities lack appropriate services and find their own means of managing waste, which has left these communities with serious environmental health risks [3].

It has been reported that the annual waste generated increased to 174 million tonnes per year in 2016 [4]. However, in 2018, only 44% received municipal solid waste collection [4]. The high volume of waste generated in SSA is attributed to rapid growth and industrialization [5]. Furthermore, projections indicate that by 2050, globally, waste will have doubled, particularly in Africa and Asia. Moreover, while waste generation continues to increase, it is reported that approximately 50% of urban waste remains uncollected [6]. In the Southern African Development Community and many other similar countries, waste management problems stem from the lack of management, high costs of service delivery, lack of infrastructure and poor enforcement from the authorities [7]. Purportedly, in rural areas, the situation is worse as the majority do not receive waste management services [8]. Hence, rural communities have resorted to alternative ways of managing waste, whereby indiscriminate dumping has become more evident, symbolizing a lack of or poor EHL [9].

Subsequently, the indiscriminate disposal of waste remains the biggest challenge in many SSA countries, as the dumping of waste, including soiled diapers, is observed along roadsides, marketplaces and other public spaces, proving this to be a common practice [10]. Subsequently, the lack of waste removal services in many rural communities in SSA countries continues to be a concern for the environment and public health [10]. These behavior indicate a lack of knowledge and environmental literacy amongst the communities. Furthermore, in a report by the United Nations International Children's Emergency Fund conducted in 2020, it was estimated that 1.7 billion people lacked access to basic sanitation services, with 494 million people practicing open defecation [11]. Open defecation is defined as the disposal of human feces in an open environment such as fields, forests, water bodies, and with municipal waste [11]. Consequently, the dumping of soiled nappies becomes a proxy of open defecation due to fecal matter found in soiled diapers that contaminates the environment.

The concept of open defecation extends to the disposal of feces contained in materials such as plastic bags, which has the potential to become exposed to the open environment irrespective of the pathway [12]. Open defecation poses a risk to environmental and public health as it is associated with the increased prevalence of diarrhea diseases, particularly in children [12]. According to the World Health Organization (WHO), diarrhea disease is the second greatest cause of mortality for children under 5 years of age worldwide, and accounts for 800,000 deaths a year primarily in the developing countries of Africa [13]. Children's fecal matter is more likely to contain enteric pathogens than adults', and open defecation by children contaminates the household environment, which may cause the transmission of diarrhea and cholera [11]. Consequently, this could happen as a result of poor or unsafe disposal of fecal waste, especially in low-income countries with fewer waste management resources. This then represents a gap in EHL [14].

2. The knowledge, attitude and behavior regarding diaper disposal in Sub-Saharan Africa

Over the last decades, there has been an increase in the global usage of disposable diapers, which was a huge transition from the use of cloth diapers [15]. Sales of nappies have grown rapidly, mostly in Africa and other Asian countries. The growth is expected to continue to increase, especially in low- middle income African countries. For instance, Nigeria is expected to see a 117% rise by 2026 [12]. Jesca et al. [16] states that there are few literature reviews offering insight into ways to handle and dispose of disposable nappies. The norm is that diapers should be rinsed off and the soils thrown into the toilet before disposal as municipal waste. However, with no specific guidelines regarding the safe disposal of diapers, hence “single use” diapers are seen polluting the environment [12].

In many SSA countries, there is a lack of monitoring, education and awareness on appropriate methods of disposing used diapers and their potential risk to the environment, as well as health risks that result from such practices [17]. These discrepancies translate to a lack of EHL, which is the ability to identify environmental health risks and apply appropriate measures to prevent any hazard [18]. Hence, the most common and safe method of disposal of solid waste utilized at household level should be done at municipal landfill sites. Subsequently, it is practiced by only a few as it is irrelevant to those in rural communities where municipal waste services are minimal, inconsistent or non-existent [4]. In addition, a survey conducted in 21 villages of Cambodia found that only 13% of care-givers used disposable diapers, even though they are considered clean, convenient and time-saving [19]. Notably, most care-givers reported that their children are taught at a very young age to use latrines, potties and other means to defecate in their yard [19]. These villages had limited access to disposable nappies because of financial income, and cloth diapers were preferred due to low cost. Subsequently, disposable diapers were found to cost three times the price of cloth diapers [14].

In contrast, the use of disposable diapers is high in other SSA countries, for instance, disposable diapers have become popular in Zimbabwe [20]. Most women use them, irrespective of the level of education, social status and age. There are different reasons to be noted in relation to why women in Zimbabwe utilize disposable diapers, namely: they were advantageous, convenient and save time, as they do not have to spend time washing [21]. It is to be noted that the women who participated in the study by Jesca et al. [16] reported using fewer nappies a day because of the ultra-absorbent material. This implied that the baby could spend several hours in one nappy. Although this was the case, their disposal was a major environmental health concern. Many areas have no system in place to cater for their disposal [22]. Furthermore, as reported, these areas lacked the capital to run the waste disposal systems efficiently. Additionally, the local authority cannot afford to provide skip bins in the communities to encourage the separation of waste at the source. Thus, people are encouraged to put disposable diapers in plastic bags and dispose of them in their bins along with municipal solid waste [17].

In Nakuru County, Kenya, 73% of care-givers dispose of soiled diapers with other household waste; 18.9% dispose of it in pit latrines; and 0.7% dispose of it in pit toilets (**Figure 1**) [23]. Also observed were caregivers’ disposing of diapers in open fields or land (**Figure 1**). Tanzania is also engulfed by similar disposal challenges, where disposable nappies contribute significantly to the waste stream generated daily by households and consumers [24]. Hence, the research estimated that this accounts for 1.5–2% of municipal solid waste and are the third largest consumer item in landfills, which represents 30% non-biodegradable waste [25]. In Tanzania, there are currently no official government statistics on the importation, handling and use of disposable diapers [24]. However, it is apparent that the use of disposable diapers has grown since the 1990s because the local standard of living and affordability has improved [26]. Consequently,

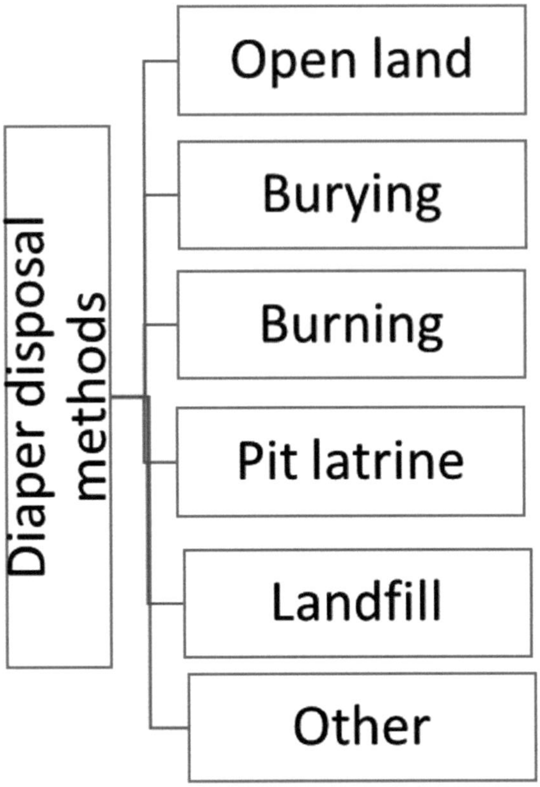

Figure 1.
Methods used for diaper disposal in rural areas.

the increased use of diapers in Tanzania's Zanzibar increases the disposal and treatment challenges for that state and the community [24].

According to Sepadi [27], 1.1 million metric tons of soiled diapers are generated and disposed of yearly in South Africa, and their usage differs from one care-giver to the next. For instance, a newborn may use 6–10 disposable diapers per day, whereas a toddler uses 3–4 diapers per day. In Mtumbane Township in the Eastern Cape, disposable diapers were found to be the second highest type of waste after food that is generated by the community. The residents at Mtumbane stored their waste in sacks, baskets and plastic bags, whilst others resorted to illegal dumping [28]. In Mthatha, Tsheleza et al. [29] found that households generated 2.84 kg/capita/week of waste and on average, solid waste generation per capita was 0.40 kg for persons living in informal settlements. Furthermore, the study found that diaper waste accounted for 17.9%, which was also the second-most type of waste generated after food waste [29]. Data collected from 19,000 sites across 82 countries between 2011 and 2018 identified disposable diapers as being amongst the top 25 most common items found in the sea, and top 40 items found in terrestrial settings, and also accounts for 21% of items found in waterways [30, 31]. Thus, these practices show a lack of education and EHL within the society.

Various methods are used to dispose of soiled diaper waste in the rural communities of SSA. The different methods of disposal are shown in **Figure 1**.

Many rural villages in SSA countries are characterized by poor waste management disposal practices, and this is causing detrimental effects on the environment. Open dumping, burying, burning of waste, pit latrines and other methods (**Figure 1**) such as using buckets to store soiled diapers are common diapers dumping practices in most developing countries [32]. Evidently, the burning of diapers causes air pollution, which further contributes to climate change because of the pollutants released into the air [33]. A common health hazard experienced by rural areas are diapers dumped in open spaces (**Figure 1**), which are often scattered by roaming dogs and cows. These diapers produce a foul smell and attract rodents and flies which can transmit diseases [34]. Similarly, disposing of diapers inside the pit latrine or burying them inside the pit hole can cause the pit to get full faster, and these could contribute to the non-sustainability of land due to diapers that cannot decompose. The improper management of waste is influenced by a lack of services, which further contributes to indiscriminate waste disposal [21]. Notably, a small percentage of rural areas dispose of waste in landfills. In according to Waste Management Standards, generated waste is supposed to be disposed of in landfill sites. However, some sites operate in open dumping sites where leachate can occur, leading to the contamination of surface and underground water [33].

Many rural communities in South Africa are living in extreme poverty, with a lack of access to basic water, sanitation, hygiene, and waste removal services [35]. Thus, the accumulation of disposable diapers in the environment is an issue. Moreover, a total of 627 disposal sites were identified and found to be near rivers. Additionally, most disposal sites were in villages where dirt roads and the grazing of animals were common [36]. These findings show that residents in rural villages see rivers as a means to wash away waste; which symbolizes lack of knowledge and literacy on environmental health risks. Consequently, indiscriminate dumping of soiled diapers may lead to the contamination of water sources with bacteria and viruses, which could contribute to health risks [36].

3. Health risk impact caused by the disposal of soiled diapers

Careless disposal of soiled diapers increases the amount of human excreta in solid waste and the environment [37]. Furthermore, it exposes people who deal with solid waste, especially municipal employees and waste pickers, to contaminants that could cause illnesses, as some may handle raw fecal matter in the process of disposing of disposable diapers [21]. This act could expose workers to different types of viruses, including enteric viruses, rotaviruses and human calici-viruses. Babies are known to be carriers of enteroviruses. Some of these pathogens have the potential to live in the excreta for several months and are likely to cause harm to people long after they have been discarded [17]. It is a health risk to handle this type of waste. It is moreover a hazard for people to handle it without being aware of its harmful effects. Hence the observation of poor waste handling in rural areas, where waste is handled without taking any precautionary measures indicate lack of EHL.

Diapers discarded in water sources and household environments may result in outbreaks of cholera, diarrheal diseases, dysentery, hepatitis A, polio and typhoid in the communities [38]. In addition, diarrheal diseases are the second leading cause of death in children, with 525,000 deaths recorded annually [39]. Similarly, cholera is an acute diarrheal infection caused by the ingestion of food or water contaminated with vibrio cholera [40], which could be spread due to fecal contamination of the environment caused by the indiscriminate dumping of soiled diapers in open land. According to WHO [40], there were approximately 1.3 to 1.4 million cases of cholera and 21,000 to 143,000 deaths worldwide due to cholera. In 2016, Zambia reported about 1179 cases of cholera, with 31 deaths, in which the most affected were children under 5 years of age [41]. Safe and sufficient water facilities and proper hygiene practices are the key to preventing not only diarrhea diseases but also acute respiratory infections [13]. Thus, it is important for communities to comprehend the appropriate measures of handling and disposing of soiled diapers.

To this end, in rural communities where waste collection is non-existent, care-givers choose to burn nappies on open land [42]. Subsequently, open burning of waste releases harmful gases and particles into the environment, which may cause potential health risks such as lower respiratory infections, lung infections and chronic obstructive pulmonary diseases [34]. Therefore, Environmental Health education and awareness on appropriate measures suitable for the disposal of diapers is important for public health gain.

4. Why care-givers use disposable diapers?

Disposable nappies have become popular in SSA countries as most women use them, irrespective of their level of education, social status and age [42]. It is observed that both working women and stay-at-home women use diapers for various reasons. Care-givers use diapers because of the advantages that they bring [43]. Most working women use diapers because they save time, as they reduce the time of doing laundry [17]. Additionally, others mentioned that they are convenient, easy to use and can be easily disposed of [18]. On the contrary, women in rural areas used diapers because of the water shortages they experience in their communities. Due to water shortages, women in rural communities sometimes spend days without water. Therefore, disposable diapers save them from dealing with foul odors that result from dirty diapers [44]. It was also discovered that some women use diapers because of their popularity and status [27]. Notably, disposable diapers use is seen as a symbol of status. Care-givers using disposable diapers of a particular brand are regarded as better off compared to those using cloth napkins [45]. Notably, it was also evident that disposable diapers were more popular amongst young women than elderly women [20]. Hence, the driving factor of disposable diaper usage is the privileged association that it brings, more than the negative impacts experienced by the environment.

Research conducted in Poland found that only 14.7% of care-givers read the instructions on diaper packages about how to use them; whilst 70% were found not to be interested in the composition of diapers [31]. This could mean that care-givers do not rinse the diaper that has been soiled by feces before disposal, posing a risk to health and the environment. Hence, there is a gap in environmental knowledge amongst the youth and the elderly in SSA countries, which is a contributing factor to waste management problems [5]. To sustain environmental issues in SSA countries, formal education for sustainable development is essential at all levels of education to elicit societal transformation. Therefore, stakeholders with the right knowledge, attitude and skills are required to educate the communities.

5. Environmental and health risk assessment process and environmental health literacy

Environmental Health literacy requires an assessment of environmental and health issues of concern as the methodology to identify if the communities and key stakeholders understand the health risks and issues within their environment and can take actions to prevent environmental degradation and health risks. Hence, the assessment process in **Figure 2** aims to identify the baseline level of EHL and measures that can be taken to implement appropriate interventions to protect health and the environment. Such action could boost the level of EHL within the community and, where needed, capacitate key stakeholder as deemed fit. The following process outlined in **Figure 2** assesses the environmental health risk assessment as the baseline for EHL, employable for an effective intervention in a typical rural community.

5.1 Step 1: Identification of environmental and health risk

This process entails identifying activities within the area and their ability to cause environmental problems or degradation that could result in health risks. In this step, one could assess environmental health risks, the related legislation and policies available to control poor environmentally degrading practices. In this step, an observation checklist can be developed to identify all areas where such activities occur. In this instance, the disposal of soiled diapers can contaminate the environment and cause health problems within the area where these activities occur, and this checklist should be able to identify all the necessary community risks aiding the problem. Communities should also be able to identify what they believe is a risk within their environment.

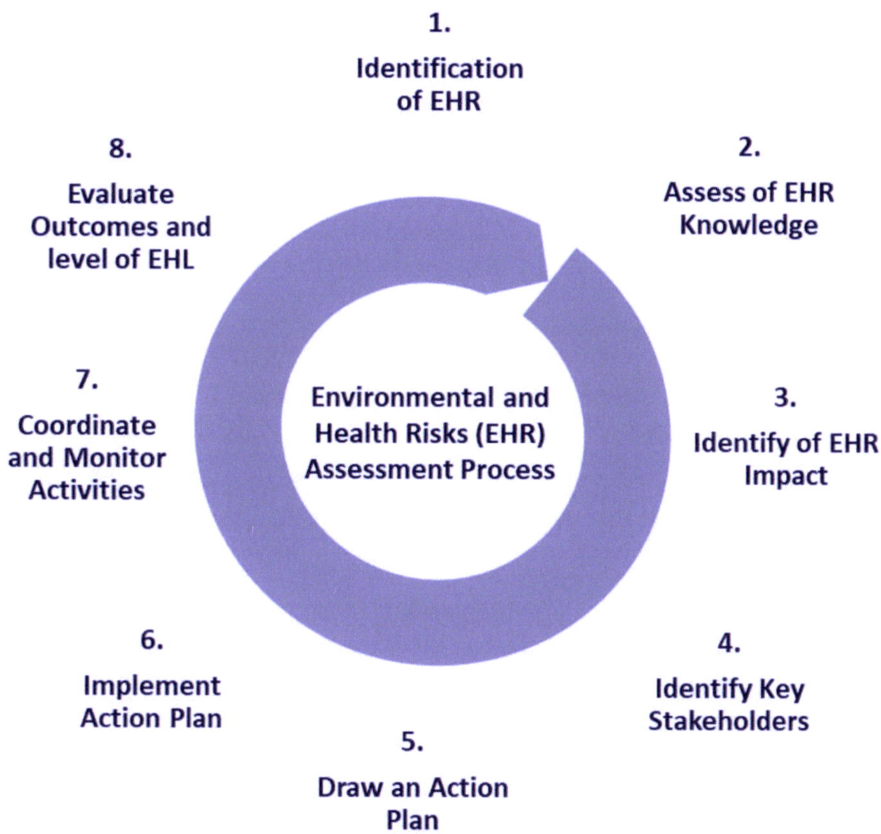

Figure 2.
Environmental health risk assessment process baseline for environmental health literacy.

5.2 Step 2: Assess environmental health knowledge

It is important to ascertain whether the communities living in the area where harmful environmental activities occur understand or know the results of environmental contamination. Communities within or adjacent to the site can be assessed through verbal interviews to determine if they know the terms of the environmental and health consequences of their actions. The checklist developed in the previous step could be useful in this process. It is also vital to determine and identify the individuals involved in activities that affect the environment and health in their area, especially indigenous knowledge in the community. Stakeholders mandated to provide services or deal with similar situations ought to be assessed to gauge their level of understanding and their available knowledge to influence the general usage of related information. These exercises will allow the assessment of the status of the EHL. The evaluation of environmental health and key stakeholders, including those involved in activities that causes problems, and the affected communities should be taken in context. The general knowledge of the community concerning the disposal of soiled diapers' effect on the environment and how it affects the communities, and everyone nearby, should be assessed. This will allow the assessor to determine if the stakeholders know what is supposed to be done to protect the environment and prevent health problems.

5.3 Step 3: Identify environmental and health impacts

Once the knowledge assessment is done, all stakeholders will be involved in identifying the environmental and health impacts. In terms of environmental issues such as the ability for community activities to contaminate the land, water resources and air, pollution will be recorded through inspection and observation. In this instance, it is known that diaper disposal on open land and burning can contaminate the environment, thereby causing land nuisance, air pollution, and waterborne diseases such as cholera and subsequently diarrhea to the consumers or end-users of such contaminated water. It must further be noted that the presence of dioxin can cause cancer after prolonged exposure.

5.4 Step 4: Identify key stakeholders

This process is essential as it identifies those key role-players and stakeholders that could provide resources. Affected stakeholders responsible for providing interventions must be identified in this step. In may be that solutions are within the abilities of other stakeholders within the community. It may be necessary that intervention decisions are taken at this step. Decision-makers could be critical as they develop policies to deal with environmental health problems. This may involve planning, implementing, monitoring and evaluating the identified outcomes of stakeholders. Similarly, communities that are affected by the behavior of those involved in poor environmental health activities should always be recorded.

5.5 Step 5: Draw an action plan

The identification of environmental and health Impacts requires a need for the development of an action plan to deal with environmental and health problems. To come up with a plan to intervene in the problem, a program needs to be set up that will include what (activity), who (affected stakeholders, i.e., Environmentalist, Health Practitioners, other interested stakeholders, individuals involved in the activities and affected communities), why (an action or activity that is causing a problem), where (the area in which such activity is taking place and the magnitude of such a problem), how (how does the activity cause an impact on the environment and health), and when (in terms of date, place and time when the intervention plan can be done).

5.6 Step 6: Implement an action plan

In this step, a target to implement the action plan developed is set. This plan should be communicated with the key participants to ensure that all stakeholders and communities that are affected participate. The message to communities must be clear and precise. Outline the benefits of intervention methods; Show the affected parties how the implementation of the action plans can lead to desirable results; and Identify the enablers that will assist to encourage the affected communities and those involved in the wrong practices of soiled disposal to voluntarily change their behavior by taking appropriate actions.

5.7 Step 7: Co-ordinate and monitor all activities

This process includes identifying all involved in addressing the common problem and assessing its mitigation strategies or activities. In this step, stakeholders should find a common way of addressing the problem to avoid conflicting messages and the duplication of services. It is important to determine how to monitor and manage conflicts amongst different stakeholders. The setting up of a monitoring strategy with goals, targets and expected outcomes is critical at this step, and this should be tied up to the monitoring of planned activities.

5.8 Step 8: Evaluate the outcomes and level of environmental health literacy

Assess if the goals, targets and outcomes are achieved. The outputs versus the outcomes in relation to the period of implementation, as well as the change observed within the environment in which communities live, are assessed. In union, the number of people in communities who are affected in terms of their health outcomes, the best practices and weaknesses are recorded. This is done to ensure that correct interventions and measures can be implemented. This step allows the assessment on the level of EHL within the communities as a baseline.

6. Conclusion

The disposal of diapers requires an understanding and proper knowledge of the risks it causes to health and the environment. Such awareness requires the communities to be aware of what it is required. This is also a complex issue as the manufacturers of these diapers do not have appropriate measures in place to protect health and the environment. Everything is left to the consumer to deal with in terms of the handling and disposal, which causes a major gap in EHL within SSA countries. Conversely, the assessment process outlined could be the first step to imparting knowledge on how to deal with diaper disposal within the communities as a method for awareness and education to improve EHL. However, the challenge experienced in SSA countries demands the need for more monitoring, education, and awareness of appropriate methods for nappy disposal. Community participation should be a cornerstone to encourage the application of appropriate waste management issues and programs required to deal with diaper disposal. In addition, clean-up campaigns should be conducted by the authorities and communities as a way of showing the negative effects of diaper disposal and sharing of appropriate knowledge. In addition, WASH programs should be conducted as they are aimed at reducing illness by improving access to safe water, sanitation and improved hygiene. Lastly, mass media should be used to disseminate information to the public as communication on the appropriate way of preventing risks that could be caused by the poor disposal of soiled diapers.

Acknowledgements

The authors acknowledge Tshwane University of Technology for the opportunity of using library resources for the study.

Conflict of interest

The authors declare no conflict of interest.

Author details

Lutendo Sylvia Mudau*, Ayanda Myranda Derby Thumbathi and Davies Veli Nkosi
Department of Environmental Health, Tshwane University of Technology, Pretoria, South Africa

*Address all correspondence to: mudauls@tut.ac.za

References

[1] Davis LF, Ramirez-Andreotta MD, Mclain JE, Kilungo A, Abrell L, Buxner S. Increasing environmental health literacy through contextual learning in communities at risk. International Journal of Environmental Research and Public Health. 2018;**15**(10):2203

[2] Doro C. Level of Knowledge on the Impact of Disposal of Baby Diapers on the Environment among Residents of Zengeza 1. Chitungwiza: BUSE; 2017

[3] Fakoya MB. Institutional challenges to municipal waste management service delivery in South Africa. Journal of Human Ecology. 2014;**45**:119-125

[4] Kaza S, Yao L, Bhada-Tata P, Van Woerden F. What a Waste 2.0: A Global Snapshot of Solid Waste Management to 2050. Washington, DC, USA: World Bank; 2018

[5] Debrah JK, Teye GK, Dinis MAP. Barriers and challenges to waste management hindering the circular economy in sub-Saharan Africa. Urban Science. 2022;**6**:57

[6] Ddiba DIW. Estimating the Potential for Resource Recovery from Productive Sanitation in Urban Areas. Stockholm, Swedan; 2016

[7] Sadc. Waste Management [Online]. 2018. Available from: https://www.sadc.int [Accessed: September 23, 2020]

[8] Seopa SHM. An Investigation of Practices and Effects of Disposable Infant Diapers on the Environment: A Case Study of Mashashane Village. Polokwane: University of Limpopo; 2021

[9] Ndlovu S, Naidoo S, Level AP. Community-Led Waste Disposal in the Umkhomazi Catchment in KwaZulu-Natal. South Africa: Joint Nature Conservation Committee; 2022

[10] Senekane MF, Makhene A, Oelofse S. A critical analysis of indigenous systems and practices of solid waste management in rural communities: The case of Maseru in Lesotho. International Journal of Environmental Research and Public Health. 2022;**19**:11654

[11] UNICEF. Water, Sanitation and Hygiene [Online]. 2019. Available from: https://www.unicef.org [Accessed: June 5, 2023]

[12] White HL, Mwapasa T, Mphasa M, Kalonde PK, Feasey N, Oliver DM, et al. Open defaecation by proxy: Tackling the increase of disposable diapers in waste piles in informal settlements. International Journal of Hygiene and Environmental Health. 2023;**250**:114171

[13] WHO. Diarrhoeal Disease [Online]. 2017. Available from: https://www.who.int [Accessed: June 4, 2023]

[14] Miller-Petrie MK, Voigt L, Mclennan L, Cairncross S, Jenkins MW. Infant and young child feces management and enabling products for their hygienic collection, transport, and disposal in Cambodia. The American Journal of Tropical Medicine and Hygiene. 2016;**94**:456

[15] Krafchik B. History of diapers and diapering. International Journal of Dermatology. 2016;**55**:4-6

[16] Jesca M, Junior M. Practices regarding disposal of soiled diapers among women of child bearing age in poor resource urban setting. Journal of Nursing and Health Science. 2015;**4**:63-67

[17] Remigios MV. The environmental health implications of the use and disposal of disposable child diapers in Senga/Nehosho suburb in Gweru City, Zimbabwe. Global Journal of Biology, Agriculture and Health Sciences. 2014;**3**:122-127

[18] Hossain S. Prospects of diaper disposal and its environmental impacts on populated urban area like Dhaka city. In: 2nd International Conference on Advances in Civil Engineering (ICACE-2014) 26-28 December 2014. Chittagong, Bangladesh: CUET; 2014

[19] Bazzano AN, Taub L, Oberhelman RA, Var C. Newborn care in the home and health facility: Formative findings for intervention research in Cambodia. Healthcare. 2016;**4**:94

[20] Kimani EW, Muchiri J, Makindi S. Soiled diapers disposal practices among caregivers in poor and middle-income urban settings. International Journal of Scientific and Research Publications. 2015

[21] Ntekpe ME, Mbong EO, Edem EN, Hussain S. Disposable diapers: Impact of disposal methods on public health and the environment. American Journal of Medicine and Public Health. 2020;**1**(2):1009

[22] Mufeyani V. Community Attitudes, Knowledge and Perceptions on Indiscriminate Disposal of Disposable Diapers in Chipadze High Density Surburb. Zimbabwe: BUSE; 2016

[23] Muia VK. Disposal methods of soiled diapers in low-income households of Nairobi County in Kenya. Journal of Applied Sciences. 2018;**4**:11-20

[24] Leaska M. Solid Waste Management of Disposable Diaper Sanitation and the Connection to Environmental Awareness for Women in Zanzibar. Independent Study Project (ISP) Collection 2441. 2016

[25] Ali N, Taib MR, Soon NP, Hassan O. Issues and management for used disposable diapers in solid waste in the city of Kuala Lumpur. Eprints.utm. 2017;7:16

[26] Mugadza S. Options for the management and recycling of disposable diaper waste in Zimbabwe's urban areas. International Open and Distance Learning Journal. 2017;**1**:34-42

[27] Sepadi MM. Unsafe management of soiled nappies in informal settlements and villages of South Africa. Cities & Health. 2022;**6**:254-257

[28] Njiva ID. The Effectiveness of Environmental Education on Waste Management Practices in Mtumbane and Maheng Townships in Port St. Johns, Eastern Cape. Kwazulu Natal: Durban University of Technology; 2018

[29] Tsheleza V, Ndhleve S, Kabiti HM, Nakin MD. Household solid waste quantification, characterisation and management practices in Mthatha City, South Africa. International Journal of Environment and Waste Management. 2022;**29**:208-229

[30] Roman L, Hardesty BD, Leonard GH, Pragnell-Raasch H, Mallos N, Campbell I, et al. A global assessment of the relationship between anthropogenic debris on land and the seafloor. Environmental Pollution. 2020;**264**:114663

[31] Płotka-Wasylka J, Makoś-Chełstowska P, Kurowska-Susdorf A, Treviño MJS, Guzmán SZ, Mostafa H, et al. End-of-life management of single-use baby diapers: Analysis of technical, health and environment aspects. Science of the Total Environment. 2022;**836**:155339

[32] Serge Kubanza N. The role of community participation in solid waste management in sub-Saharan Africa: A study of Orlando east, Johannesburg, South Africa. South African Geographical Journal. 2021;**103**:223-236

[33] Rabaji OP. Waste Dumping in Sharpeville (Emfuleni Municipality): An Investigation of the Characteristics and the Potential Impacts on Air Quality. South Africa: North-West University; 2019

[34] Mathe M. Environmental pollution-perceptions and views on usage and disposal of diapers: A case study of Gwanda urban. Environmental Pollution. 2018;**3**

[35] Haywood LK, Kapwata T, Oelofse S, Breetzke G, Wright CY. Waste disposal practices in low-income settlements of South Africa. International Journal of Environmental Research and Public Health. 2021;**18**:8176

[36] Kordecki H, Antrobus-Wuth R, Uys M-T, van Wyk I, Root ED, Berrian AM. Disposable diaper waste accumulation at the human-livestock-wildlife interface: A one health approach. Environmental Challenges. 2022;**8**:100589

[37] Ochelle A. Status of Used Diapers Disposal in Githurai Ward, Roysambu Sub-County, Nairobi County, Kenya. Kenya: Kenyatta University; 2021

[38] Kusumawati D, Mangkoedihardjo S. Promising approach for composting disposable diapers enhanced by cyanobacteria. Global Journal of Environmental Science and Management. 2021;**7**:439-456

[39] Lochoro GA. Occurrence and Factors Associated with Childhood Diarrhea in Namalu Sub-County, Nakapiripirit District. Uganda: Makerere University; 2020

[40] WHO. Cholera [Online]. 2022. Available from: https://www.who.int [Accessed: June 5, 2023]

[41] Sambo J, Muchindu M, Nyambe S, Yamauchi T. Sustainable solid waste management an assessment of solid waste treatment in Lusaka, Zambia. Sanitation Value Chain. 2020;**4**:39-50

[42] Tembo E, Chazireni E. The negative environmental impact of disposable diapers: The case of Mberengwa District, Zimbabwe. International Journal of Healthcare Sciences. 2016;**4**:2158-2161

[43] Khoo SC, Phang XY, Ng CM, Lim KL, Lam SS, Ma NL. Recent technologies for treatment and recycling of used disposable baby diapers. Process Safety and Environmental Protection. 2019;**123**:116-129

[44] Nyamayedenga VK, Tsvere M. Real time data capture: A response to unsustainable dumping of disposable diapers and sanitary pads in Gweru City, Zimbabwe. East African Journal of Education and Social Sciences (EAJESS). 2020;**1**:54-64

[45] Khanyile A, Caws GC, Nkomo SPL, Mkhize NM. Characterisation study of various disposable diaper brands. Sustainability. 2020;**12**:10437

Chapter 7

Perspective Chapter: Affordance-Based Reverse Engineering of Natural Systems

Dominic Halsmer and Domenica Baez

Abstract

Affordance-based Reverse Systems Engineering (ARSE) focuses on the key enabling relationships between elements of a complex system (part-to-part affordances), and the enabling relationships between the system and its end users (end-user affordances). A novel application of this methodology to natural systems assists in a deeper understanding of the issues surrounding biological evolution, and the critical role of those precursor systems upon which it depends for success. ARSE represents an objective approach to these important questions since affordances simply delineate what actions the elements of a complex system, including the end user, can potentially take. Life-related systems are characterized by dependent sequences of affordances that are both spatially and chronologically nested across a broad spectrum of scientific disciplines. A reverse engineering approach that attends to all these sequences contributes to a more philosophically satisfying retrodiction in applying abductive reasoning to both the human condition and the cosmos as a whole.

Keywords: reverse engineering, systems engineering, affordance, natural systems, teleology, design detection, biological evolution, philosophical cosmology

1. Introduction

Can scientists, philosophers and engineers cooperate to gain insight into the mysteries of the human condition? Danish philosopher Søren Kierkegaard is purported to have said, "Life can only be understood backwards; but it must be lived forwards [1]."[1] Thus is summarized the great challenge of the human condition: To apply the *present* knowledge of our existence in deciphering the mysteries of our *past* (retrodiction) in order that we might proceed wisely into our *future*. The issues that swirl around the

[1] The actual quote is "It is really true what philosophy tells us, that life must be understood backwards. But with this, one forgets the second proposition, that it must be lived forwards. A proposition which, the more it is subjected to careful thought, the more it ends up concluding precisely that life at any given moment cannot really ever be fully understood; exactly because there is no single moment where time stops completely in order for me to take position [to do this]: going backwards." (Translation from Danish by Palle Jorgensen. Available from: https://homepage.math.uiowa.edu/~jorgen/kierkegaardquotesource.html [Accessed: March 23, 2023]).

riddle of human origins deserve careful consideration, since the question of how we proceed is not uncoupled from the question of how we came about. These questions are big enough to enlist the services of multiple academic disciplines, especially the sciences, and the humanities, but also engineering.

The sciences are fundamental to our understanding of physical reality. And the humanities lie at the heart of comprehending human existence. But the practitioners of these approaches to truth-seeking have found it challenging to work together in addressing such big questions [2]. However, engineers find themselves in the unenviable position to serve as natural mediators between the sciences and the humanities. Engineering is concerned with applying the discoveries of science to address the needs and desires of the human population. This may normally involve the (forward) engineering design of some practical widget. But we propose that engineers have a further role to play by addressing some of these bigger questions, especially when it comes to implementing the concept of reverse engineering.

Reverse engineering has been defined as "the process for discovering the fundamental principles that underlie and enable a device... or system through the systematic analysis of its structure and, if possible, its function and operation. Usually, it involves taking the aforementioned apart and analyzing its makeup and workings... part by part... until the entire entity has been analyzed and is understood [3]." Reverse engineering is most often applied to gain understanding of artificial (humanly engineered) systems. But for many years now the biological sciences have had great success when bringing a reverse engineering approach to bear on living systems. Biologist E. O. Wilson claimed that "the surest way to grasp complexity in the brain, as in any other biological system, is to think of it as an engineering problem... Researchers in biomechanics have discovered time and again that organic structures evolved by natural selection conform to high levels of efficiency when judged by engineering criteria [4]."

As evolutionary biology has matured, a fresh appreciation for more complex environmental interactions has emerged. A new Extended Evolutionary Synthesis (EES) has been developed to account for the effects of niche construction, epigenetics, and "large-scale reengineering of the genome in response to environmental stimuli," in addition to a number of other influences [5]. This renewed focus on interactions between the organism and its environment naturally leads to the concept of (end-user) affordances, defined as the organism's enabling (or disabling) relationships with various aspects of the environment.

The authors submit this work as a continuation of an ongoing effort to synthesize discoveries and approaches from multiple disciplines that bear on the big questions associated with the human condition. We strive to objectively apply a reverse systems engineering approach with a focus on affordances, as described below. While a completely objective approach may be impossible to attain, we attempt to recognize our prejudices (i.e., monotheism) and eliminate irrational bias as much as possible.

2. Reverse systems engineering with a focus on affordances

Gestalt psychologist Kurt Koffka first suggested the usefulness of affordances in the early twentieth century. He asserted that humans perceive affordances in nature, culminating in the idea that things "tell us what to do with them." He continued, "Each thing says what it is...a fruit says 'Eat me'; water says 'Drink me'; Thunder says 'Fear me'; and woman says 'Love me' [6]." Though Koffka's litany possesses a certain romantic flair, a more egalitarian perspective recognizes the preeminence of this most powerful of human affordances to *all* people; As the ancient Jewish proverb says, "What a person desires is unfailing love [7]."

But it was psychologist James Gibson who sharply advanced this concept by applying it to the field of ecological psychology in his seminal work, "The Theory of Affordances [8]." He claimed that affordances can be positive (enabling) or negative (disabling) and that they might be hidden from the senses. As in Koffka's example, a body of water affords the quenching of thirst (hydration), as well as swimming, but it also affords drowning! especially in the case of a hidden undertow that sometimes occurs at the beach. More recent researchers have explored the connections between affordances and niche construction [9]. emphasizing the idea that "affordances are not mere action possibilities but that they can also invite behavior [10]."

Don Norman, with degrees in both psychology and engineering, introduced the concept of affordances to the field of engineering with his book *The Design of Everyday Things*. In an engineering context, he clarified that "An affordance is a relationship between the properties of an object and the capabilities of the agent that determine just how the object could possibly be used;" adding that "Affordances provide strong clues to the operation of things [11]." His reference to affordances as "clues" provides an early indication of their value for reverse engineering. Another early adopter of this idea was computer scientist William Gaver who asserted, "Affordances should be useful in exploring the psychological claims inherent in artifacts and the rationale of designs [12]." He further explored the idea of hidden affordances in more complex systems, introducing the concept of "sequential affordances... to refer to situations in which acting on a perceptible affordance leads to information indicating new [previously hidden] affordances." He continued, "Sequential affordances explain how affordances can be revealed over time; nested affordances describe affordances that are grouped in space...The role of a good interface [between engineered system and end-user] is to guide attention via well-designed groups of sequential and nested affordances [13]." The identification of these different types of interdependent affordances is vitally important when conducting reverse *systems* engineering on complex systems consisting of multiple interacting subsystems.

But the engineering researcher who has most thoroughly explored the potential of affordances for assisting with both engineering design and reverse engineering is undoubtedly Jonathan Maier. He refers to affordance-based design as a "relational theory for design" since it helps to "explain the entanglement between designers, users, and [engineered] artifacts [14].[2] He has also proposed "an affordance-based method for reverse engineering and redesign [15]." This approach involves the careful analysis of an existing system "to see how it works and could possibly be improved [16]." Maier contends that after identifying and evaluating the affordances at every level, a system has been effectively reverse engineered in the sense that its operation should be well understood [17]. The reason affordances are so enlightening is because they exhibit complementarity. That is, they are relational in a way that illuminates

[2] Furthermore, affordance-based design and affordance-based reverse engineering are inherently relational at the most fundamental level since affordances are defined to be relationships, either between the end-user and the system, or between parts of the system. Maier appears to have extended the definition of affordances to include the part-to-part variety. Some researchers have objected to this extension. Even so, these part-to-part interactions (to use an alternate term) appear to play a vital role in ultimately bringing the end-user affordances into existence. For this reason, engineering researchers have found the extension quite helpful. And no disrespect to the field of ecological psychology is intended.

how two things fit together in allowing for a potential outcome, be it positive or negative [18]. But the emergence of a particular affordance does not necessarily imply that the outcome is enabled to a high degree. Thus, affordances also exhibit quality, which describes how well the system affords a particular outcome [18].

Maier refers to the triad of (1) engineer, (2) engineered system, and (3) end-user of the system as the "big picture" of engineering design. He claims that a careful consideration of the relationships between all three entities is important for successful engineering design, and affordances help to capture these interactions [19]. In extending this approach to reverse engineering, the authors have introduced a fourth component to fully capture all six of the important interactions within the big picture of reverse engineering (see the double arrows in **Figure 1**, adapted from ref. [20]). This fourth entity is the investigator of the existing engineered system, or the "reverse engineer." Several examples that help to clarify this approach are described in the first author's recent book, *Hacking the Cosmos* [21]. A classic example from the twentieth century is the reverse engineering of the Antikythera Mechanism, delightfully recounted by Jo Marchant in her book, *Decoding the Heavens* [22]. From this account, we learn that reverse engineering projects draw, not only from the sciences, but also from history, culture, philosophy and any other pertinent knowledge base. This will prove true for natural systems as well. In the case of the Antikythera Mechanism, the engineered system was (it is no longer intact) an ancient, but highly advanced astrolabe, parts of which were recovered from a shipwreck off the coast of the Greek island of Antikythera in 1900 CE. The designer is the person (or persons) who devised and built the mechanism around 100 BCE. The end-user was the person (or persons) for whom it was originally engineered; those who operated the mechanism in the years after it was built; presumably for educational purposes, or perhaps as a status-symbol. And the investigator (or reverse engineer) is the group of scientists and engineers who spent the better part of the twentieth century attempting to unravel the mysteries of this most captivating device. As one can imagine, attending to the relationships between these four entities, which leads to several interesting affordances, has the potential to lend great insight into any reverse engineering project.

When dealing with more complex systems, a useful analysis tool for "concept exploration and attention directing" has been developed, known as the Affordance Structure Matrix (ASM) [23]. This instrument lists the system components across the top of the array (columns) and the resulting affordances along the side (rows). Populated elements of the array indicate which system components interact to produce end-user and part-to-part affordances. Both positive and negative affordances are included to assist in either engineering design or reverse engineering

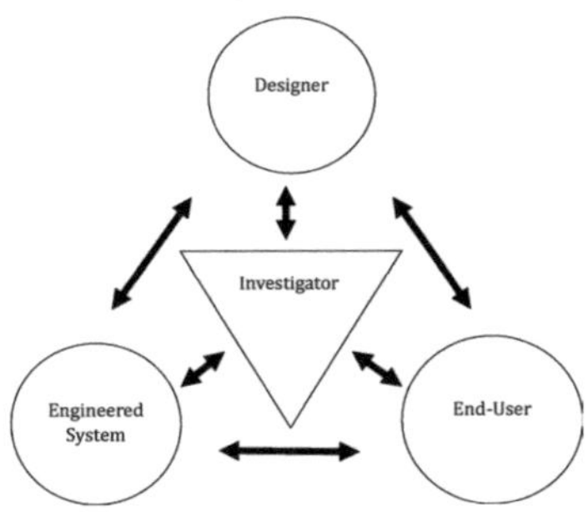

Figure 1.
The "Big Picture" of reverse engineering involves six relationships.

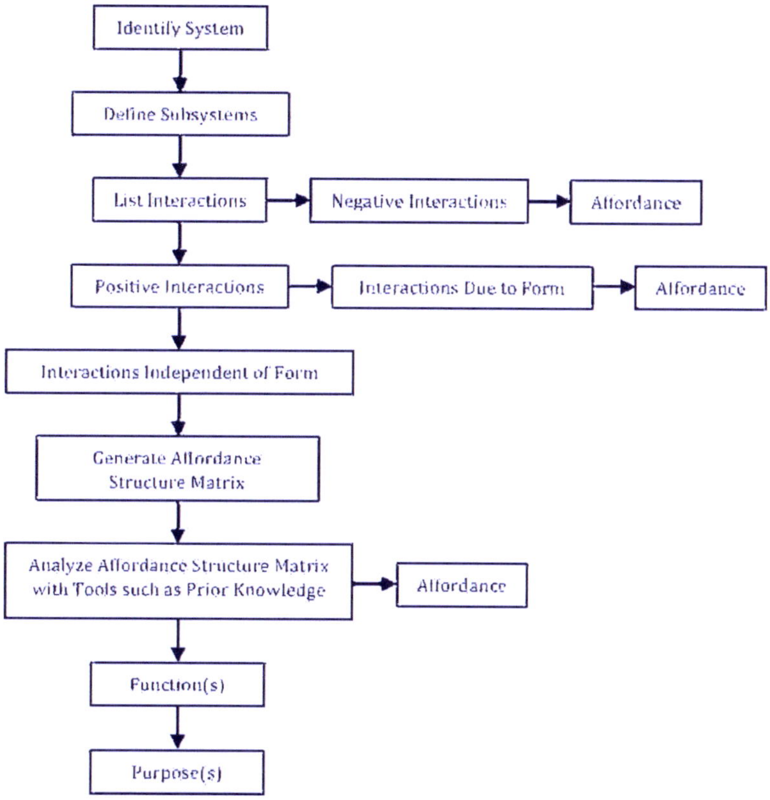

Figure 2.
Flowchart for affordance-based reverse engineering.

and redesign. In either case, the goal is to choose and arrange system components to maximize the number and quality of positive affordances and minimize the number and liability of negative affordances. Minor modifications have sought to improve the effectiveness of this two-dimensional layout by applying relative weightings to the affordances [24, 25]. Many examples of ASMs can be found in the references [14–19]. In addition, a flowchart has been developed to illustrate a step-by-step procedure for conducting affordance-based reverse engineering (see **Figure 2**, adapted from ref. [20]). Affordances are identified as component interactions are analyzed at the system and subsystem levels. An affordance structure matrix is very helpful in this process. Now let us consider the application of this approach to gain a deeper understanding of natural systems.

3. Application of ARSE to natural systems

3.1 Justification and a comprehensible Cosmos

Reverse engineering is rightly applied to artificial, or human-made systems. But one might doubt the legitimacy of applying this approach to natural systems, even in the face of reverse engineering's recent successes in biology. It may seem "unnatural" to think and speak in teleological terms when analyzing living organisms, much less inanimate objects such as water and rocks. But recent work in the philosophy of science suggests otherwise. Gunnar Babcock argues for the legitimacy of speaking in teleological terms of inanimate objects if we see that their function comes from a larger goal [26]. He makes use of McShea's field theoretic account of teleology which states that external fields are responsible for the teleology of a system. These fields direct the entities within them persistently and plastically. Persistence refers to the tendency of a system that is following a certain pattern to keep repeating that pattern, while plasticity is the propensity of a system to choose a specific trajectory from several different starting points.

For example, if we put a ball in a bowl, it will always tend to fall toward the center because of the action of gravity. Even if the ball itself has no internal program that forces it to move to the center, we can still talk about its teleology if we consider that it has functionality as part of the system of gravity and that it still deviates slightly from its course depending on its starting point. All objects can have some level of teleology, and the higher their degree of persistence and plasticity, the higher their teleology. Hurricanes exhibit these characteristics since they generally appear in the same region but will change course according to atmospheric conditions. As another example, we observe a kind of natural selection in eroding rocks, since harder rocks survive over softer rocks during erosion processes. Geologists hypothesize that mineral species over Earth's history have evolved with the changing environment. Various higher-level fields of temperature, pressure and biological interactions are responsible for the great variety of minerals we have today [26].

But how can humans even make sense of nature? We take for granted our unique ability to unravel the deep mysteries of the cosmos. Multiple advantageous circumstances have contributed to our technological understanding and advancement. Firstly, although natural systems are often incredibly complex, they exhibit extensive repeatability and generally follow orderly laws. In addition, the ordering of matter and energy, and the laws of nature are readily and accurately described by abstract entities and operations known as mathematics, which are somehow apprehended by the minds of scientists and engineers. Furthermore, human beings appear to be particularly well-suited and often highly motivated to decipher the secrets of the universe. They are especially successful in this pursuit when they make good use of all the tools at their disposal, and their efforts are remarkably profitable for humanity [20]. Indeed, the Earth, and all of nature, seems to be laid out in such a way as to facilitate scientific discovery [27, 28]. Albert Einstein recognized the significance of this match between human mental capacity and cosmic complexity (a prerequisite for reverse engineering) when he famously remarked that the most incomprehensible thing about the world is that it is comprehensible [29].[3]

[3] Einstein's actual words provide a deeper understanding of his perspective, and belie an appreciation for the importance of *relations* (or affordances) in comprehending the universe:

"The very fact that the totality of our sense experiences is such that by means of thinking (operations with concepts, and the creation and use of definite functional *relations* between them, and the coordination of sense experiences to these concepts) it can be put in order, this fact is one that leaves us in awe, but which we shall never understand. One may say, 'The eternal mystery of the world is its comprehensibility.' It is one of the great realizations of Immanuel Kant that the postulation of a real external world would be senseless without this comprehensibility".

In speaking here of 'comprehensibility,' the expression is used in its most modest sense. It implies: the production of some sort of order among sense impressions, this order being produced by the creation of general concepts, *relations* between these concepts, and by definite *relations* of some kind between the concepts and sense experience. It is in this sense that the world of our sense experiences is comprehensible. The fact that it is comprehensible is a miracle." (emphasis added).

The development of powerful microscopes has assisted in reverse engineering on the smallest scales. The chemical elements of our Periodic Table now provide the building blocks (like Lego blocks) and part-to-part affordances for the flourishing of nanotechnology. Biochemist Michael Denton alludes to the similarity between atoms and Legos as he writes, "The total number and diversity of possible chemical structures that may be constructed out of carbon, oxygen, hydrogen, and nitrogen is virtually unlimited. Almost any imaginable chemical shape and chemical property can be derived. Together these elements form what is in effect a universal chemical constructor kit [30]." Furthermore, the semi-permanent combinability of these elements appears to be absolutely reliable. We can count on certain reactions to always take place under a given set of conditions. This order and reliability at the foundation of the material world is actually a very remarkable feature of the cosmos, which was not fully recognized until the field of chemistry had sufficiently matured. Cosmologist Helge Kragh describes the impact this discovery had on the great scientist James Clerk Maxwell: "He [Maxwell] was impressed by the fact, as revealed by the spectroscope, that molecules of the same chemical species were all alike and had not changed the slightest 'since the time when Nature began.' Uniformity in time as well as uniformity one-to-another strongly indicated that atoms and molecules were created... Borrowing an expression from John Herschel, he famously (and with an allusion to natural theology) referred to the molecule as a 'manufactured article' [31]."

Philosopher Richard Swinburne points out that "any theory that at a beginning or always there were many substances, which fall into kinds with identical powers and liabilities, is again a theory of a very improbable coincidence." He continues, "Such a coincidence cries out for explanation in terms of some single common source with the power to produce it. Just as we would seek to explain all the coins of the realm having an identical pattern in terms of their origin from a common mould, or all of many pictures having a common style in terms of their being painted by the same painter, so we should seek to explain all physical objects having the same powers in terms of their deriving them from a common source [32]." With these and other arguments, Swinburne attempts to mathematically quantify the question of God's existence based on the natural world, and concludes that it is at least as likely as not. Quite simply, the universe appears to be the work of some kind of cosmic engineer (or engineers), as incredible as that sounds. Like the proverbial onion, the events of our expanding cosmos portray layer upon layer of nested affordances that ultimately lead to planet Earth and the life that so curiously flourishes upon it. Given the connection between affordances and engineering,[4] it seems warranted to take an affordance-based reverse engineering approach to understanding natural systems. Such an approach may only be an exploratory hypothesis to be evaluated based on the success it engenders. But the authors consider that the tentative application of ARSE across the entire realm of nature seems justified by the evidence up to this point.[5]

[4] Basically, engineers use their knowledge of science and mathematics, along with their own ingenuity and resourcefulness, to create end-user affordances for their customers. This typically involves the clever arrangement and layering of nested part-to-part affordances within a system, device, or product. This type of affordance structure is what is found in nature, but in the extreme.

[5] While the authors currently maintain a theistic worldview, this perspective is open to revision based on the pertinent evidence from all fields of knowledge. We endeavor to be objective in our approach and seek to eliminate irrational bias as much as possible, while acknowledging the difficulty in completely avoiding all egocentric and sociocentric thinking [33].

3.2 Objectivity and the affordances that enable evolution

Maier argues that affordances represent an objective approach to understanding natural systems since they simply describe what can occur within such a system and what actions an end-user can potentially take. This leads to a common terminology and mutual understanding by people with very different worldviews. He writes, "[In reverse engineering of biological systems,] the function/purpose of any system is inherently subjectively defined. For example, while an evolutionist may not say that the *function* of a brain is to think,[6] while a creationist would certainly say that it is, they could both agree to the fact that brains *afford* thinking [34]." Philosopher John Sanders agrees with Maier and argues further for the foundational nature of affordances. He claims that affordances "offer a conceptual tool of exceptional value in the construction of a positive theory of embodied agency [i.e., humanity], and of its philosophical consequences [35]." He asserts that affordances "deserve to be given a leading role in...first philosophy [36].[7] "Why should affordances enjoy such a prominent place in understanding reality? Sanders writes, "while ontology [the study of being] must be relativized to what different observers can do in terms of affordances, this is no mere matter of what the observer *thinks* or *believes*. It is a function of what the observer *can do*, and this may be as objective a matter as anyone could hope [37]." In short, an affordance relationship simply results in an undeniable enablement that is independent of various philosophies or beliefs involving function or purpose.

But even if a single affordance is free of teleological baggage, the picture is not as clear when groups of affordances are found in nested layers that appear to ingeniously provide opportunities of great value, such as human life and love. Could these kinds of affordance structures be signs of a deeper reality? In thinking specifically about human perception of affordances as signs, psychologist John Pickering writes that, "The characteristic reflexivity of human cognition means that we are not only able to perceive the world as it is,...but also to perceive affordances that do not yet exist, that is, to perceive the world as if it were otherwise...and hence we may take meaningful, intentional action to bring it about if we so choose." He adds that, "nature is a harmonious sign system," implying that affordances are signs that are indicative of meaning and purpose in the world. Thus, affordances appear to be critically important for studying "the interactions of animals, plants and their surroundings [which] are the concern of biosemiotics, the study of natural signs [38]." Renowned physicist George Ellis takes a similar perspective as he recently proposed the introduction of "possibility spaces" into the sciences. He writes, "I claim that the deep structure of the universe is timeless, eternal *possibility spaces* of a Platonic nature. These underlie the nature of what is possible in the physical universe and what is not... These are a way of re-expressing the nature of the laws of physics in terms of a space of possible physical outcomes [39]." In other words, his possibility spaces represent what can be in the universe and what agents can think and do in the universe, which arise directly from part-to-part and end-user affordances.

When seen in the light of nested affordances, the success of biological evolution depends on a long and complex series of dependent precursor relationships, both internal and external to living organisms. Biologist Christian de Duve said it well:

---

[6] Most evolutionists would be averse to this language since it evokes teleological thinking reminiscent of a designer.

[7] "First philosophy" deals with the fundamental type of being or substance upon which all others depend, and with the most fundamental causes.

"[Evolution] did not operate in a vacuum. It operated in a universe governed by orderly laws and made of matter endowed with specific properties. These laws and properties are the constraints that shape the evolutionary roulette and restrict the numbers that can turn up [40]." His reference to laws and properties could be stated more generally in terms of affordances that determine what is biologically possible in the universe. In considering the preconditions for biological evolution, a helpful resource is Philosopher Rope Kojonen's recent book, *The Compatibility of Evolution and Design*. Kojonen evaluates reasons for the common assumption that evolution and design are competing explanations, and develops an alternate view. In the fourth chapter (Not by Selection Alone: Evolutionary Explanations and Their Requirements) he explores the intriguing aspects of nature upon which evolution depends. In reference to an entire evolutionary pathway, he writes, "...it is not clear whether the direction taken by the evolutionary series as a whole is impacted by other factors beyond those that we can discern in an isolated evolutionary event. The possibility of accumulating these mutations and forming new forms of life might still require other factors, such as the existence of an environment that supports the existence of this kind of form, the existence of natural selection, and the existence of a functional series of intermediate steps that connect functional forms. If such preconditions play a substantial role in making evolution possible, then this also needs to be taken into account in constructing the picture of evolution as a whole, and how it relates to design arguments. Supposing that these preconditions are the result of design, then it would no longer be true that evolution proceeds without design [41]."

But is there evidence to suggest that these preconditions are the result of design? Kojonen lays out affirmative reasoning, but biology is complex and only a few of his arguments are briefly summarized here. Regarding recent work to develop genetic algorithms (computer programs) to simulate the creative ability of evolution, he writes, "...it does seem credible to conclude that in genetic algorithms, the production of new information does depend on the existence of prior information in the system, and that such algorithms can only solve problems that they are specifically designed to solve. The systems must be built to reward stepwise growth, and the selective conditions must be adapted to the problem being solved. Thus, in these simulations, the possibility of evolution depends on design, demonstrating that there is no necessary contradiction. One can further argue that due to the strong dependency of the algorithm on design, the products of the simulated evolutionary process are revelatory of the intelligence of the programmer [42]." Some biologists, such as Denton, have adopted a "structuralist" view of evolution in which biological forms are the consequence of the laws of physics and chemistry, merely discovered by evolution. Such "laws of form" describe how relationships between elementary forms might ultimately afford more complex forms, as addressed by Kojonen: "In order for evolution to be possible, viable forms must be close enough to each other in the space of possible forms, and must form a network that can be navigated by evolutionary search. The study of protein evolution and convergence, among other factors, provides evidence that the course of evolution is directed by the structure of the space of forms, as well as laws of form, arising as a consequence of the laws of physics. Also, it may be that evolutionary biology could be understood as even hospitable to teleological interpretation, once all elements of the extended synthesis are considered fully [43]."

To be sure, the extended evolutionary synthesis more fully recognizes the key impact of relational interactions between organisms and environments (end-user affordances), and appears to more fully appreciate the pre-existing relationships that led up to and nurtured evolutionary processes (sequential and nested part-to-part affordances). The term "fine-tuned" has become popular in referencing the universe's apparent fitness for life, but the authors believe a more accurate term is "engineered." Indeed, the fact that natural systems are so readily and profitably reverse engineered by humans strongly suggests that these systems were engineered in the first place [44]. The connectedness of everything in the universe (heavily laden with affordances [45]) is aptly described in the following quote by the famous naturalist, John Muir, "When we try to pick out anything by itself, we find it hitched to everything else [46]." As part of his conclusion to chapter four, Kojonen writes, "The more our understanding of evolution has progressed, the more we find ourselves explaining patterns in evolution by reference to general principles, rather than just contingent historical events (which continue to have a great role in all models). Instead of explaining the appearance of purpose in biology by reference to non-teleological factors, the attempt at explaining design by evolution has succeeded in finding new layers of teleology. The further we study, the more the universe seems to be filled with teleology 'all the way down!' [47]". The authors contend that an understanding of natural affordances, with the methodology introduced in this paper, helps to clarify our conception of the natural world, and assists in the formulation of a philosophically satisfying worldview. This approach is illustrated further in the following example involving life on planet Earth.

3.3 Example: A planet teaming with life

As expressed in the introductory section, we ultimately want to gain a better understanding of the origin and fundamental nature of human beings. Perhaps the knowledge gained will afford us the ability to act with more wisdom in the future. This goal suggests that humans be chosen as the natural system of study in this example application of ARSE. But as stressed above, human evolution cannot be effectively studied in isolation from the surrounding Earth environment, including all other living organisms. Indeed, we now know that the development of life on earth depended on the part-to-part affordances inherent in the processes of stellar evolution and the early expansion of the universe.[8] Thus, a more comprehensive approach might choose the entire cosmos as the natural system of study. Though a bit excessive for this paper, it is the topic of the first author's recent book, *Hacking the Cosmos*. Thus, the authors have settled on planet Earth and its life forms (focusing on humans in particular) as the natural system of study for this example.[9]

Even so, it is very challenging to apply ARSE to something as massive and complex as planet Earth and all its inhabitants. But the advantage of reverse *systems* engineering is the ability to break things down into subsystems and subsequently smaller modules. This will certainly be necessary as we proceed with this example, but to clarify the playing field at the outset, the place to start is with the big picture of reverse engineering shown previously in **Figure 1**. And a good place to start in the big picture is with the engineered system: planet Earth and the life it supports. In thinking about the designer (or original engineer) of this system, an atheist might choose to leave this spot vacant, while a theist would be comfortable with a supernatural deity (or deities)

[8] The chemical elements necessary for life (as we know it) arose out of the hellish conditions within stars during stellar nucleosynthesis. And the conditions that led to stellar nucleosynthesis arose from the interesting interplay between the influences of gravity and dark energy in the moments after the big bang.

[9] Of course, the sun, moon and nearby planets will need to be included as well since they obviously influence the possibility and development of life on Earth.

of some kind. Because it aligns with the beliefs of a large segment of the population and leads to some interesting philosophical considerations, for this example, we will hypothesize a Maker[10] consistent with the traditional (Abrahamic) monotheistic religions. In filling the role of end-user, we are tempted by our anthropocentrism to insert ourselves. But we must remember that we are not the only inhabitants that enjoy the affordances associated with life on Earth. And it appears that all the participants in the web of life are important for life to flourish. Furthermore, a Maker of the aforementioned tradition is believed to have made all things for divine purposes. So for theists, there is a sense in which the Maker is not only the designer, but the ultimate end-user. This brings us to the final player in the reverse engineering quartet: the investigator (or reverse engineer). In this case, the reverse engineer is anyone who is curious and sincere enough to honestly delve into the deep mysteries surrounding how and why life is thriving on planet Earth. From where did life come? How did it originate and progress? How do we explain the extreme positives and negatives of the human condition? And is there a deeper meaning and purpose to life that should guide our actions?

A few general words should also be offered regarding the relationships between the four entities that make up the big picture of reverse engineering. While the designer of an engineered system would typically have in-depth and complete knowledge of the system, the end-user might only possess operational knowledge of the system; enough to use it effectively (or perhaps misuse it), without understanding every technical detail. However, an active relationship between the user and designer, including information exchange about the system, should lead to more effective and successful use of the system. The same is true for the reverse engineer, who would certainly seek out information exchange with the designer (if possible), or any documentation the designer might offer regarding the system. But the curiosity of the reverse engineer would typically take them deeper than operational knowledge of the system. This deeper knowledge could also be passed back to users to enhance their experience of the system. In the case of our living planet, scientists and other educators admirably perform this role. In considering the human condition on Earth, one of the most puzzling paradoxes is the great potential and hope users typically sense for a happy and successful life, which is so often met with commonly experienced negatives such as confusion, disappointment, disease, personal failure, and despair.[11] This state of affairs serves to lead some users into the role of reverse engineer as they strive to enhance their understanding of reality. Users/reverse engineers should also consider the possibility that this need for additional information (beyond that which is inherent to the system) might be made available in a different kind of knowledge format. Indeed, it makes sense that a good Cosmic Engineer (if one exists) would provide such additional communication to users if needed. This kind of helpful knowledge might come in the form of divine revelations, sacred writings, or incarnations.[12]

[10] The term "Maker" was intentionally chosen (as opposed to Creator) to maintain openness to the manner in which this Cosmic Engineer made the Earth and its inhabitants.

[11] And the big one, which is death. What is the point of life if it all ends after a few years on Earth? Indeed, many people believe there is compelling evidence for an eternal and fulfilling afterlife that commences after the physical body passes away.

[12] Although these forms of knowledge certainly go beyond the realm of science, they are not necessarily anti-scientific. As mentioned earlier, all pertinent areas of knowledge should be explored when conducting reverse engineering studies.

The next step in the ARSE methodology is the systematic identification of affordances by literal and/or figurative dissection of the system. After identifying the Earth as the system (following the flowchart in **Figure 2**), important subsystems are defined. We know that the Earth is a dynamic combination of interacting subsystems that have been changing over long time periods. Thus, layers of nested and sequential affordances are identified as (enabling or disabling) relationships occurring over both space and time. The simplest initial decomposition breaks the "Earth system" into four major spheres (hydrosphere, atmosphere, geosphere, and biosphere). However, "the interactions among Earth's four spheres are incalculably complex [48]."

Even so, fundamental affordances are recognized in the relationship between the hydrosphere and the biosphere: for example, living organisms experience life-sustaining *hydration*. Similarly, the atmosphere affords life-sustaining *aeration* to the biosphere, as well as the *mitigation* of potentially life-threatening solar radiation and *protection* from the harsh cold of space. Through the action of gravity, the large mass of the geosphere affords a *dwelling* place for the other three spheres, which allows for their close interaction in space. For example, hydration is further enabled by the global water cycle, in which close interaction and exchange occur between the hydrosphere, atmosphere and geosphere, with obvious benefit to the biosphere. But along with the rain comes the potential for flooding in the valleys and dangerous debris flows in the mountains, with obvious disabling influences. Thus, negative affordances such as *inundation* and *drowning* are also recognized. Many more affordances could be identified, especially as the four Earth spheres are further broken down into additional subsystems. In addition, the sun, moon, and nearby planets exact their influences on the Earth and its inhabitants, illuminating even more affordances...But space is limited, so our discussion thus far will have to suffice.

A simple Affordance Structure Matrix (See **Figure 3**, adapted from ref. [20]) helps to illustrate how some of the subsystems and components interact resulting in affordances, but it is obviously far from exhaustive. In this ASM, the biosphere has been further subdivided into plants, animals, and humans. These, as well as a few other important components of the system, are shown across the top of the matrix. Significant end-user (EUA) and part-to-part (PPA) affordances are listed down the left side. The filling of the matrix then indicates which components contribute to which affordances. For example, the water cycle results from interactions among the four Earth spheres and the sun. Although life is listed as a positive end user affordance, it is also the result of many layers of a myriad of sequential and nested part-to-part affordances, hence the contributions from all system elements. This type of high-density affordance structure is characteristic of engineered systems.

Though a helpful indicator of component participation (see totals to the right), the ASM is not a very effective tool for representing the sequential and nested hierarchical dependencies of affordance structures. Perhaps a more helpful representation is the dependency graph, which is used extensively in the development and reverse engineering of computer software and systems. A dependency graph simply shows the directional dependencies of several objects toward each other. Software engineer Winston Ewert has proposed the dependency graph as a new hypothesis to explain the nested hierarchical patterns associated with living organisms. He conducted an extensive quantitative analysis and concluded that "The biological data was a better

		hydrosphere	atmosphere	geosphere	sun	moon	stars	plants	animals	humans	total
+EUA	Life	x	x	x	x	x	x	x	x	x	9
	Education	x	x	x	x	x	x	x	x	x	9
	Loving Actions							x	x	x	3
-EUA	Pollution	x	x	x	x	x		x	x	x	8
	Evil Actions							x	x	x	3
	Drowning	x								x	2
+PPA	Water Cycle	x	x	x	x			x	x	x	7
	Rock Cycle	x	x	x	x			x	x		6
	Stable Spin Axis			x	x	x					3
-PPA	Earthquakes	x		x	x	x					4
	Birth Defects							x	x	x	3
	Asteroid Strikes			x	x	x	x				4
	total	7	5	8	8	6	3	8	8	8	61

Figure 3.
Simple affordance structure matrix (ASM) for life on earth. EUA: end-user affordance; and PPA: part-to-part affordance.

fit to a dependency graph than to a tree [structure] [49],[13] ultimately suggesting that DNA was constructed by a process similar to the automated compiling of a computer code [50].

On a larger scale, a simple dependency graph has been developed to illustrate the dynamic structures related to the evolution of the cosmos and living organisms from the origin of the universe (see **Figure 4**). Only the main pathways are shown, and many details have obviously been omitted for space and clarity, but it demonstrates the numerous layers of sequential and nested affordances that underlie planet Earth and its inhabitants. The emergence of a complex life form that can not only perform marvelous engineering feats, but also look back and marvel at the ingenuity with which they were engineered, is certainly a very curious development. Indeed, the whole realm of nature provides inspiration for humans engaged in the practice of engineering, as is evident from the biomimicry revolution [51]. Gaining knowledge

[13] Ewert explains further, "The dependency graph is essentially a tree with extra flexibility; the modules can explain genes shared between species thought to be only distantly related by common descent. A module is not restricted to reusing code from a single source, but can freely reuse from multiple sources. Compare this to common descent where each species must almost exclusively draw from a single source: its ancestral species." (p. 3).

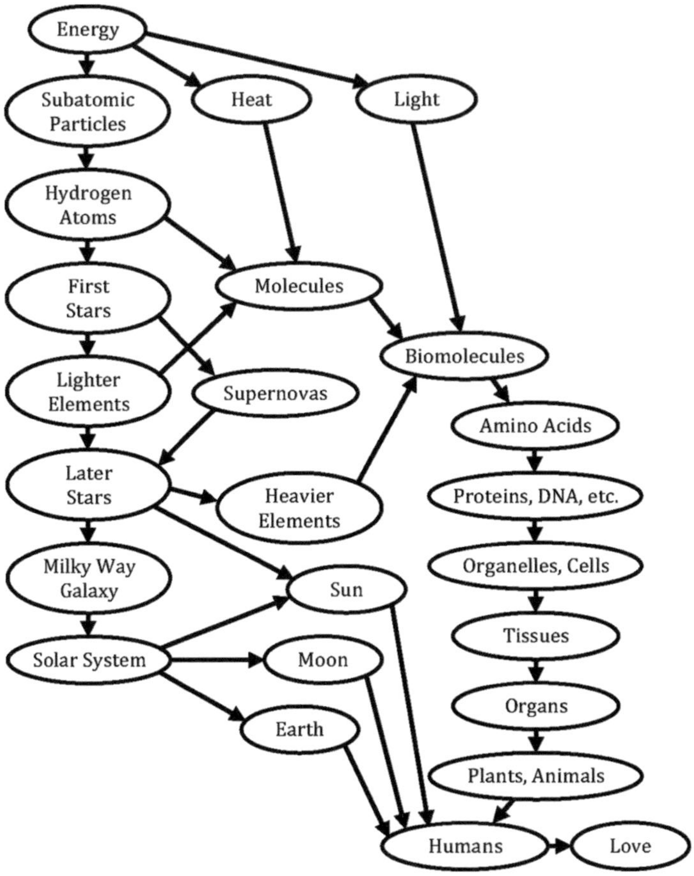

Figure 4.
Simple dependency graph for earth and its life forms.

and wisdom from nature is the key idea of biomimetics, both to better care for the Earth, and to better understand our own nature as humans.

4. Summary and conclusion

Incorporating the concept of affordance (and extending it to include part-to-part interactions) into reverse systems engineering has led to a novel methodology of exploration, which has been fruitfully applied to enhance our understanding of both natural and artificial systems. While individual affordances objectively describe what can occur in a system, multiple layers of sequential and nested positive affordances are indicative of function and purpose. Investigating all the relationships in the big picture of reverse engineering and considering the pertinent evidence from all knowledge bases is especially important. ARSE appears to be an effective methodology for hacking the planet and advancing our understanding of the human condition. However, this approach is only as good as the models that are developed to represent reality. Thus, the ARSE methodology is limited by the difficulty of capturing all the important relationships along with their associated consequences.

The system of life on planet Earth offers an intriguing example in abductive reasoning. The emergence and development of living organisms depends on long strings of sequential and nested affordances that point to some kind of Cosmic Engineer, even in the face of significant evidence for biological evolution. Indeed, the very preconditions on which the evolutionary paradigm depends for success seem to have been engineered to ensure that success. In this sense, evolution and design appear to be quite compatible, as Kojonen suggests. Even so, the substantial negatives of the human condition offer a sobering check to this idea. But in light of the hope that we somehow persist beyond the grave, perhaps these negatives form a necessary part of the system; one that affords real freedom to complex organisms, training in the ability to fully love, and the apprehension of vital truths; truths that become ever clearer as we continue the quest of hacking the cosmos! [52].

Acknowledgements

I am grateful to all the students and faculty at Oral Roberts University who assisted me in this research over the last several years.

Conflict of interest

The authors declare no conflict of interest.

Author details

Dominic Halsmer and Domenica Baez*
Oral Roberts University, Tulsa, OK, United States

*Address all correspondence to: dhalsmer@oru.edu

References

[1] Kierkegaard S, Journalen JJ. Søren Kierkegaards Skrifter. Vol. 18. Copenhagen: Søren Kierkegaard Research Center; 1997. p. 306

[2] Kegan J. The Three Cultures: Natural Sciences, Social Sciences and the Humanities in the 21st Century. Cambridge: Cambridge University Press; 2009. DOI: 10.1017/CBO9780511576638

[3] Messler RW. Reverse Engineering: Mechanisms, Structures, Systems and Materials. New York: McGraw Hill; 2014. p. 16

[4] Wilson EO. Consilience: The Unity of Knowledge. Westminster, MD: Knopf Publishing Group; 1992. p. 112

[5] Garte S. New ideas in evolutionary biology: From NDMS to EES. Perspectives on Science and Christian Faith. 2016;**68**(1):3-11

[6] Koffka K. Principles of Gestalt Psychology. Vol. 7. New York: Harcourt, Brace and World; 1935. p. 353. DOI: 10.4324/9781315009292

[7] The Holy Bible, New International Version. The Committee on Bible Translation, Zondervan; 1973. Proverbs 19:22

[8] Gibson J. The theory of affordances. In: Shaw RE, Bransford J, editors. Perceiving, Acting and Knowing. Hillsdale, NJ: Erlbaum Associates; 1977. pp. 67-82

[9] Withagen R, van Wermeskerken M. The role of affordances in the evolutionary process reconsidered: A niche construction perspective. Theory and Psychology. 2010;**20**(4):489-510. DOI: 10.1177/0959354310361405

[10] Withagen R, de Poel H, Araujo D, Pepping G. Affordances can invite behavior: Reconsidering the relationship between affordances and agency. New Ideas in Psychology. 2012;**20**:250-258. DOI: 10.1016/j.newideapsych.2011.12.003

[11] Norman D. The Design of Everyday Things. Revised and Expanded ed. Vol. 11. New York: Basic Books; 2013. p. 13

[12] Gaver WW. Technology affordances. In: CHI '91 Proceedings of the SIGCHI Conference on Human Factors in Computing Systems. New York; 1991. p. 83. DOI: 10.1145/108844.108856

[13] Gaver WW. Technology affordances. In: CHI '91 Proceedings of the SIGCHI Conference on Human Factors in Computing Systems. New York; 1991. p. 82. DOI: 10.1145/108844.108856

[14] Maier JRA, Fadel GM. Affordance based design: A relational theory of design. Research in Engineering Design. 2009;**20**(1):13. DOI: 10.1007/s00163-008-0060-3

[15] Maier JRA, Fadel GM. Affordance based design methods for innovative design, redesign and reverse engineering. Research in Engineering Design. 2009;**20**(4):225. DOI: 10.1007/s00163-009-0064-7

[16] Maier JRA, Fadel GM. Affordance based design methods for innovative design, redesign and reverse engineering. Research in Engineering Design. 2009;**20**(4):234. DOI: 10.1007/s00163-009-0064-7

[17] Maier JRA. Affordance Based Design: Theoretical Foundations and Practical Applications. Saarbrucken, Germany: VDM Verlag; 2011. p. 84

[18] Maier JRA, Fadel GM. Affordance based design: A relational theory of design. Research in Engineering Design. 2009;**20**(1):21. DOI: 10.1007/s00163-008-0060-3

[19] Maier JRA. Affordance Based Design: Theoretical Foundations and Practical Applications. Saarbrucken, Germany: VDM Verlag; 2011. pp. 41-61

[20] Halsmer D, Roman N, Todd T. Integrating the concept of affordance into function-based reverse engineering with application to complex natural systems. In: Proceedings of the Annual Conference of the American Society for Engineering Education; 14-17 June 2009, Austin TX. Washington, DC: ASEE; 2009

[21] Halsmer D. Hacking the Cosmos: How Reverse Engineering Uncovers Organization, Ingenuity and the Care of a Maker. Dubuque IA: Kendall Hunt; 2019. pp. 109-134

[22] Marchant J. Decoding the Heavens: A 2,000-Year-Old Computer – And the Century-Long Search to Discover its Secrets. Cambridge, MA: Da Capo Press; 2009

[23] Maier JRA, Ezhilan T, Fadel GM. The affordance structure matrix – A concept exploration and attention directing tool for affordance based design. In: Proceedings of the ASME International Design Engineering Technical Conferences and Information in Engineering Conference IDETC/CIE; 4-7 September 2007; Las Vegas, NV. New York: ASME; 2007. DOI: 10.1115/DETC2007-34526

[24] Maier JRA, Sandel J, Fadel GM. Extending the affordance structure matrix – Mapping design structure and requirements to behavior. In: Proceedings of the 10th International Design Structure Matrix Conference DSM'08; 11-12 November 2008, Stockholm, Sweden. New York: ASME; 2007, 2008

[25] Maier JRA, Sachs R, Fadel GM. A comparative study of quantitative scales to populate affordance structure matrices. In: Proceedings of the ASME International Design Engineering Technical Conferences & Computers and Information in Engineering Conference IDETC/CIE; August 30–September 7, 2009; San Diego, CA. New York: ASME; 2009. DOI: 10.1115/DETC2009-86524

[26] Babcock G. Teleology and function in non-living nature. Philosophical Science Archives. 2023;**201**(4):1-20. DOI: 10.1007/s11229-023-04099-1

[27] Gonzalez G, Richards JW. The Privileged Planet: How our Place in the Cosmos Is Designed for Discovery. Washington, DC: Regnery; 2004

[28] Wiker B, Witt J. A Meaningful World: How the Arts and Sciences Reveal the Genius of Nature. Downers Grove, IL: InterVarsity; 2006

[29] Einstein A. Ideas and Opinions. New York: Crown; 1954. p. 292

[30] Denton M. Nature's Destiny: How the Laws of Biology Reveal Purpose in the Universe. New York: Free Press; 1998. p. 108

[31] Kragh H. Matter and Spirit in the Universe: Scientific and Religious Preludes to Modern Cosmology. London: Imperial College Press; 2004. p. 35. DOI: 10.1142/p338

[32] Swinburne R. The Existence of God. Oxford: Oxford University Press; 2004. p. 164. DOI: 10.1093/acprof:oso/9780199271672.001.0001

[33] Paul R, Elder L. The Miniature Guide to Critical Thinking: Concepts and Tools.

Tomales, CA: The Foundation for Critical Thinking; 2009. pp. 21-22

[34] Maier JRA. Affordance Based Design: Theoretical Foundations and Practical Applications. Saarbrucken, Germany: VDM Verlag; 2011. p. 166. (emphasis in original)

[35] Sanders JT. Affordances: An ecological approach to first philosophy. In: Weiss G, Haber HF, editors. Perspectives on Embodiment: The Intersections of Nature and Culture. New York: Routledge; 1999. p. 122

[36] Sanders JT. Affordances: An ecological approach to first philosophy. In: Weiss G, Haber HF, editors. Perspectives on Embodiment: The Intersections of Nature and Culture. New York: Routledge; 1999. p. 136

[37] Sanders JT. Affordances: An ecological approach to first philosophy. In: Weiss G, Haber HF, editors. Perspectives on Embodiment: The Intersections of Nature and Culture. New York: Routledge; 1999. p. 133 (emphasis in original)

[38] Pickering J. Affordances are signs. tripleC. 2007;5(2):64-74. DOI: 10.31269/triplec.v5i2.59

[39] Ellis G. The Philosophical Problems of Cosmology. IAI News [Internet]. 2021. Available from: https://iai.tv/articles/the-philosophical-problems-of-cosmology-auid-1883?_auid=2020 [Accessed: April 04, 2023]

[40] Giberson K, Artigas M. Oracles of Science: Celebrity Scientists Versus God and Religion. Oxford: Oxford University Press; 2006. pp. 32-33

[41] Kojonen EVR. The Compatibility of Evolution and Design. Cham, Switzerland: Palgrave Macmillan; 2021. pp. 103-104. DOI: 10.1007/9783030696832

[42] Kojonen EVR. The Compatibility of Evolution and Design. Cham, Switzerland: Palgrave Macmillan; 2021. p. 113. DOI: 10.1007/9783030696832

[43] Kojonen EVR. The Compatibility of Evolution and Design. Cham, Switzerland: Palgrave Macmillan; 2021. p. 132. DOI: 10.1007/9783030696832

[44] Halsmer D, Halsmer N, Johnson R, Wanjiku J. The applicability of engineering design principles in formulating a coherent cosmology and worldview. In: Proceedings of the Annual Conference of the American Society for Engineering Education; 22-25 June 2008; Pittsburg, PA. Washington, DC: ASME; 2008. DOI: 10.18260/1-2--3501

[45] Rietveld E, Kiverstein J. A rich landscape of affordances. Ecological Psychology. 2014;**26**(4):325-352. DOI: 10.1080/10407413.2014.958035

[46] Muir J. My First Summer in the Sierra, Sierra Club Books. 1988th ed. Boston: Houghton Mifflin; 1911. p. 110. DOI: 10.5962/bhl.title.19229

[47] Kojonen EVR. The Compatibility of Evolution and Design. Cham, Switzerland: Palgrave Macmillan; 2021. p. 133. DOI: 10.1007/9783030696832

[48] Lutgens FK, Tarbuck EJ. Foundations of Earth Science. 8th ed. Upper Saddle River NJ: Pearson; 2017. p. 8

[49] Ewert W. The dependency graph of life. BIO-Complexity. 2018;**3**:18. DOI: 10.5048/BIO-C.2018.3

[50] Ewert W. The dependency graph of life. BIO-Complexity. 2018;**3**:5. DOI: 10.5048/BIO-C.2018.3

[51] Dicks H. The Biomimicry Revolution: Learning from Nature How to Inhabit the Earth. New York: Columbia University Press; 2023. DOI: 10.7312/dick20880

[52] Halsmer D. Hacking the Cosmos: How Reverse Engineering Uncovers Organization, Ingenuity and the Care of a Maker. Dubuque IA: Kendall Hunt; 2019